Mastering
NLP YOGA
Now

WAYNE CHUNG

KIRIN INTERNATIONAL A.G.

Master the NLP Yoga Now
All Rights Reserved.
Copyright © 2017 Wayne Chung
v1.0

The opinions expressed in this manuscript are solely the opinions of the author and do not represent the opinions or thoughts of the publisher. The author has represented and warranted full ownership and/or legal right to publish all the materials in this book.

This book may not be reproduced, transmitted, or stored in whole or in part by any means, including graphic, electronic, or mechanical without the express written consent of the publisher except in the case of brief quotations embodied in critical articles and reviews.

KIRIN INTERNATIONAL A.G.

ISBN: 978-0-578-19234-5

Library of Congress Control Number: 2017941609

Cover Photo © 2017 thinkstockphotos.com. All rights reserved - used with permission.

PRINTED IN THE UNITED STATES OF AMERICA

ABOUT THE WRITER

Wayne Chung is a youthful, energetic, loving, confident and responsible business coach and personal coach from Hong Kong. Wayne Chung is also a financial service practitioner. Out of his vast and in-depth practice, Wayne Chung founded ALLIED MERCANTILE BANK CORPORATION (SWIFT CODE: ALMRMPMP), a few futures commercial merchants, Introducing Brokers (FCMs/IBs) worldwide, and an international trust company.

Wayne Chung, a master practitioner in NLP and the WH Method, completed brilliant studies in Philosophy of Mind, Bhagavad Gita, Philosophy of Yoga and Puranas from Oxford University. Wayne Chung earned MSc in Financial Management in 1998 and BSc (Hons) Economics in 1996 in London. Wayne Chung is currently studying political science with London School of Economics and Political Science. He is a frequent business traveler as well as traveling for societal improvements on different continents.

Wayne Chung has assisted many high net worth individuals (HNWI) and high net worth corporations (HNWC) from China,

Hong Kong, Thailand, Indonesia, Malaysia and Singapore to set up corporate wealth structure as well as private wealth structure and observed that successful personalities can be modeled. He shows others also how to start and run a new bank or futures/forex trading company, private wealth structure, corporate structure or offshore company-related matters, Wayne Chung can be reached at wolverhampton@offshoredragon.com. For subconscious mind matters, please use nlpyoga@offshoredragon.com

ACKNOWLEDGEMENTS

I have too many people to thank, who have all supported me and cared about me in my private life and my roles as householder, financial engineer, tax consultant, banking and finance practitioner, trust administrator, charity worker and NLP Yoga practitioner. This book is dedicated to all of you I've met along the path at different times. You are awesome!

"NLP" refers to "Neuro linguistic programming" which was originally created by Richard Bandler and John Grinder in the 1970s. Basically, NLP is using the language of the brain via a system of methods and techniques to assist in replacing negative habits, limiting beliefs, mental blocks and fears with new supporting beliefs. Yoga is a group of physical, mental, and spiritual practices or disciplines which may involve stretching.

Ms Christine Chow
Assistant Registrar
for Registrar of Trademarks
Singapore

06 October 2016

BAHAYA / DANGEROUS/危険/ κίνδυνος / опасность / והנכס/ 위험

NLP Yoga is a powerful operational manual of human behaviors that is made easy. It can transform you into a stronger individual. You may bypass reading and stop practicing NLP Yoga should you be complacent with your present state, values and belief system, because NLP Yoga is full of vibrancies, positivities, energies, activities, resources, people networks, possibilities and loves which extend beyond your present frontier. Therefore, the author highly suggests that you read and understand the front and rear cover of the book again and take responsibility for your own actions based on what you are going to learn from the content of NLP Yoga. Flipping past this page signifies your tacit acknowledgment of the power of NLP Yoga.

TABLE OF CONTENTS

Preface i

About this book v

1. Operating Manual 1

2. Accumulators/Minibonds Movement 4

3. Are you Ready for the Main Course? 10

4. The AMWAY Movement 12

5. The Neuro-linguistic Programming Movement 19

6. The Fire within Bhagavad Gita 41

7. The Meaning of Yoga 55

8. The Contemporary/Modern Yoga Movement 57

9. Pre NLP Yoga 72

10. Yoga in the Bhagavad-gita 82

11. How to blend NLP into Yoga and vice versa? 125

12. NLP Yoga : Know it, Use it 142

13. Appendix. 143

14. The Seven Main Teachings of Bahagavad Gita. 227

PREFACE

What to expect from this book

This book, the NLP Yoga that you are holding in your hands now is combined and becomes NLP, Yoga, and Bhagavad Gita explained in plain but empowered words. Yes, you are acquiring two most powerful skillsets in human life simultaneously. Living the NLP Yoga way, you won't need to divert your attention to unproductive chores in all aspects of your life but you can stay focused upon your best productive activities. Just do it, for it is very possible. For those who need further coaching and perhaps an NLP Yoga retreat, please contact bhakti@nlpyogin.com .

NLP Yoga is an awakening process, ascension and a kind reminder to prepare you to exceed any previous cognitive limitations of all that you think you are lacking. You are about to let go of old limited beliefs, values, ideas about who you are, how you feel about yourself, what you say to yourself during solitude and how you sound. You are moving toward increasing your energy and developing yourself to live an empowered life from this very moment.

I am confident, I can do it. Yes!!

MASTER THE NLP YOGA NOW

By extracting certain proven presuppositions and application tools from NLP, Yoga and Bhagavad Gita, NLP Yoga provides you with everything you need right now to tap into your own power to create greater excellence and live an empowered life. If you would like to make your life meaningful and achieve your goals more swiftly, then you are about to discover the secrets from this book.

Every action begins with imagination in your head. First, you must know your desired outcome and take action. Take real action—not aiming, aiming, and forever aiming. Pay attention to your results, both good ones and those for which you need feedback. The results should provide the most honest feedback that you can collect from all sources. Be willing to change your action, behaviors and take fresh action again and again. Always focus on excellence, not perfection, as almost nothing is perfect. This is an expansive way to live your life and provides you with a simple set of strong foundations upon which you can improve in all aspects of your life, i.e. health, wealth, relationships, career, business, etc.

NLP Yoga is all about reliable and valid guidance for you to take charge of your mind--to consciously set your subconscious mind to work the best for you. Have you ever realized that it is not what you do not know that hinders your growth (e.g. a career promotion, business tender, etc). It has more to do with the knowledge that you possess which is untrue! People tend to store intellectual knowledge that is not productive or providing growth as the brain does not differentiate between good or bad. The human brain works like a rubbish bin if you use it like that. Therefore, this is time to unlearn some knowledge and habits that no longer serve your needs.

ABOUT THIS BOOK

Since the civilization of mankind, yogis are always tagged as achievers of the highest state among mankind. Many people all over the globe are fanatical about learning yoga for various motivations that their instructors claim, e.g. health, sexual attraction, etc. Speaking of the highest state of yogi, your mind may form a picture of a blue-colored man with long hair and skin lotion of mud and ash, with eyes closed as he sits on tiger skin. You are seriously warned that the meaning of information generated from pictures in your mind could be simply your own interpretation of what you've perceived from external sources. Release your mind from the yogi picture and come back to earth. Accuracy and precision in sciences, mathematics, astrology, medicine and technologies, etc during ancient periods are still being discussed today in respective fields of study by world class academicians and professionals. Do you know that most of the greatest scientists during that time were yogis (also known as yogin or enlightened sages)? Do you also know that there are hardly any average people in this world? For example, according to the World Bank the GDP per capita in the USA during 2013 was USD53,041.98. Ask yourself and ask those around you and record the number of people in the USA who earned that amount of money during that period of time. The answer is that a majority of the people in the USA didn't earn that amount of money during 2013. Therefore, do not try to become an average person, it is much harder of a struggle than you could imagine if you attempt to become one. This is such a cruel book because it reveals more significant knowledge in greater detail. It is absolutely up to you whether you want to learn all it takes to become a yogin personality or an average personality.

The secret of success of yogin is meditation or what is also known as yoga practice on mind, or mind training. It is not the purpose of this book to prove or enter into debate on the origin of yoga. It was recorded in the authoritative ancient text, the Bhagavad Gita (the Gita) that the Master of Yoga revealed His teaching of various yoga systems during the dangerous wartime on the Kurukshetra Battlefied in India 3000 BCE some 5,000 years ago. More than a proven by time 'philosophy,' the teachings in the Gita are a set of operating manuals for achievers and leaders. The Gita is the place of origin of law of karma, law of attraction, law of nature, law of self and the law of universe. Master these laws with NLP Yoga and you achieve the personality of greater excellence.

The ability of the Gita to reveal the most fundamental of all wisdom has been admired by Albert Einstein: "When I read Bhagavad Gita and reflect about how God created this universe, everything else seems so superfluous." That's right, the greatest scientist believed in the God in the Gita.

ABOUT THIS BOOK

History repeats itself. Gain and pain from the past can reappear in just a matter of time. Otherwise who is going to spend time and money to record the history and require someone else to pass the exam paper of history? Important knowledge and wisdom will absolutely gain weight over time. The Gita has been an influential text and growing more widely studied in the United States of America. To name a few, Harvard Business School students are reading the Gita (http://www.dnaindia.com/mumbai/report-harvard-students-studying-the-gita-ramayana-univ-president-1640315). Forbes 500 CEOs are reading the Gita (http://www.forbesgroup.com/inner2.iml?mdl=articles.mdl&ArticleID=43&ArticleCat=2). In addition to that, during November 2008, Seton Hall University, a private Roman Catholic university in South Orange, New Jersey, United States made the study of the *Gita* mandatory for every student attending the university. Lately, Grade 5 students in the Netherlands also study the Gita (http://www.tamilbrahmins.com/showthread.php?t=32677). The Gita is a must read text for people of all age groups and NLP Yoga made the reading of Gita more enjoyable and productive. The earlier you start to read and practice NLP Yoga, the more benefits you achieve. The Gita is a 700-verse Hindu scripture in Sanskrit that is part of the Hindu epic *Mahabharata* (chapters 25 - 42 of the 6th book of Mahabharata).This is the right time to learn Gita's Yoga-based NLP to create excellence in your personality and let NLP Yoga coach you along your way in acquiring this highest knowledge. It is safe to learn the Gita.

I am confident, I can do it. Yes!!

During the 1970s, there was another operating manual for modeling achievers and leaders through programming language communicating to the human brain, neuros and body. This operating manual is called Neuro-Linguistic Programming (NLP). There are some similarities as well as gaps between the two great operating manuals for creating excellence in personality, namely Gita-spoken Yoga and NLP. NLP is result-action (nearly but not exactly Karma Yoga) driven. Gita spoken Yoga is result-focus-realized knowledge-action (Bhakti Yoga-Dhyana Yoga-Jnana Yoga-Karma Yoga) driven. NLP Yoga discovered that NLP actually practices some of the useful philosophies and techniques presented from the Gita either unconsciously or with some variations. Therefore, it is important for those who are interested in NLP or already practicing NLP to gain a deeper understanding and practice of the Gita teaching.

Your mind may have wondered what cocktail-like effect would occur when the operating manual of 5,000 years ago was brewed with the contemporary NLP operating manual. The purpose of this book is not to replace any NLP Yoga practice. I know that you already agreed that NLP Yoga practice is very important for you and you must start learning, practicing and mastering NLP Yoga immediately. However, you must perseveringly put in a lot of serious effort and totally immerse yourself in NLP Yoga now to achieve your greatest success even though you may enjoy the fruit or nectar of success of the NLP Yoga at a very early stage. Do not be complacent with early results. Do not pluck the fruits prematurely; work on it persistently and this is the only guarantee and assurance that you will keep on creating greater excellence in your personalities one after another. As long as you practice NLP Yoga diligently, success is always the only product and the byproduct, isn't it?

Instead of integrating NLP and Yoga blindly to come out with a commercial program, NLP Yoga studies the NLP and Yoga techniques and common motivations of all human beings - happiness, prosperity, abundance, health, peace of mind, positivity, etc. in short, dreams and realizations of dreams. Some of these dreams are derived from the domain of materials and some are from the domain of spirituals. In the world of NLP Yoga, dreams are achievable.

In this book, NLP Yoga presents observations on a few contemporary and important international movements which really changed and influenced mankind for learning and sharing purposes. You will neither find any judgmental views imposed on these observations nor does NLP Yoga give any hindsight financial analysis. Instead, NLP Yoga wants you to see for yourself how sociology and psychology, NLP and Yoga work congruently and you find out the root cause of why you must seriously master NLP Yoga after reading this book. We will never solve any problem effectively at surface level unless we reach the root cause, face it and solve it. NLP Yoga hope you enjoy reading this book and go all-out to share what you would have learned regarding NLP Yoga earlier with your loved ones.

OPERATING MANUAL

Before you buy a machine/home appliance/electric item/vehicle etc, you first ask for an operating manual to learn how to duly use the item that you are about to purchase. This is to make sure that you understand and know how to use it purposefully, safely, effectively, ecologically, wisely. This is the most important step that you must undertake no matter how much the salesperson has convinced you to consider buying. Of course, you can also obtain third party opinions on the operating manual. Users will find some operating manuals written on a product which has gone through comprehensive research and development and testing, with proven, reliable and valid results. Before you instruct your body to achieve some result, have you ever first found out who you are, what you really want, and how to give effective instruction to your body to act? Huh? I knew some of you did ask your parents or guardians when you were younger and your search for feedback was not satisfied.

Do human beings improve themselves better with or without consciously following an operating manual? The answer is that you must consciously use the operating manual. Great world athletes, sportsmen, singers, actors, politicians, speakers, contenders, etc. have all operated by a strict manual whether through rapid/immersed training or simply being especially gifted. Operating manuals are sometimes also known as protocols/disciplines/menus/formulas/faculties/prescriptions/rituals/recipes. One must be trained regarding how to use the operating manual to achieve efficacy in the desired outcome.

If you do not operate yourself with a competent operating manual, your neurons, brain, behaviors and actions can be easily hacked and hijacked by others who are operating with a higher version and more powerfully neuro-linguistic operating manual. Advertisement hijacks the audience's operating manual by converting their buying behavior, doesn't it? Every single human being is functioning with his or her own operating manual either consciously or unconsciously.

Sages and Yogin adhere strictly to their operating manuals consciously. I know you are already asking for contemporary and real life examples. Before you turn to the next chapter, please do this exercise:

1. Find a comfortable place and sit down with your spine and head straight. Close your eyes take a deep breath through your nostrils, flow the air throughout your body from the neurons head to toes and toes to head a few times to as many times as you can and pay attention to your inhalation, the entire flow of air and then exhale.

2. Now go back to the most recent time when you felt most motivated in your life. Put yourself into your body during that time. Feel what you felt. Hear what you heard. Smell what you smelled. See what you saw.

3. Open your eyes, stand up. Shake your body harder!

4. Repeat Step 1 above. Ask yourself what operational manual you were operating by when you were highly motivated (the same event in Step 2 above). Aries, Taurus, Gemini, Cancer, Leo, Virgo, Libra, Scorpio, Sagittarius, Capricorn, Aquarius or Pisces?

Whatever answer it is, starting from this moment you will be the master of your own personality and operate with your own tailor-made and unique operating manual. You will manifest your qualities internally and externally to create all the excellence that you want in your life. People who do this exercise before turning to the next page will benefit multiple times more than those who choose to skip this. Get a timer or someone to keep track of the time for you. Fifteen minutes is most effective. This is the only exercise in this book.

ACCUMULATORS/ MINIBONDS MOVEMENT

Let's have some starters before the main course. Soup?Salad?Hong Kong dim-sum? Singapore's chili crab? Near the beginning of the 21st century, the neurons of mainly Chinese investors from Hong Kong, Singapore and mainland China were programmed to swing from one extreme to another. Many high net worth investors, professional investors, and even institution investors (http://www.wsj.com/articles/SB122460075958054287) were victimized by the famous banking product called '"Accumulator" (Hong Kong accent pronounces it as "I kill you later") through some highly educated, specially trained beautiful-looking private bankers and licensed wealth managers. If you look at the product name and the sales channel (http://www.ft.com/cms/s/0/ce9028ba-e9b8-11dd-9535-0000779fd2ac.html#axzz4K38usjfh) at the surface level, you may be led to believe that this must be some premium quality wealth accumulation solution only affordable for the high net worth or simply the rich. If the victims of "accumulator" bothered to look at the root makings of the product before adding their signatures on the agreement, they should have avoided this financial crisis of the century.

In brevity, accumulators are structured financial products. By entering into an accumulator contract, you are agreeing to purchase a fixed amount of financial instruments (i.e. security, commodity or currency) from a bank on a daily basis at a predetermined price **("strike price")**. The contract usually lasts for a year, i.e. 250 trading days. The strike price is set at a specified percentage of the initial market price of the financial instrument **("initial spot price")** so as to enable buyers to accumulate the financial instrument at a discount. If the price of the financial instrument rises to 3%- 5% above the Initial spot price, the contract will be knocked out and the investor is under no obligation to follow through on the contract. However, if the price of the financial instrument goes below the Strike Price, the contract will continue and investors are obliged to keep accumulating the underlying financial instrument, notwithstanding that they are buying shares at a loss. After the wild crash of financial markets worldwide during the Lehman Brothers scandal, the prices of many stocks reached their year's lowest, and it became unlikely that the stock prices would rise to a level that would trigger a knock-out before the expiry of the accumulator contracts. Thus some investors chose to square off their open positions on accumulation contracts to cut losses, which inevitably attracted a significant penalty.

Therefore, accumulators are very risky products not suitable for non-risk takers. The investor's gain is capped at a certain level but the extent of his losses is not limited. The downside risk seems remote when the market is good, but once the risk is realized the consequences can be disastrous. This is especially the case for investors who leveraged their accumulator contracts on credit margin; these investors ended up losing all their money and owed large sums of money to banks. Accumulator at its root is a financial derivative product that can push investors into over-loss (losing more than their investment capital). Also, Lehman's mini-bonds weren't bonds at all. The name was linguistically programmed to inspire confidence in the product, but in reality they were credit-linked notes assembled using complex derivatives. Most developed markets, including the USA and UK, prohibit the sale of these notes to retail investors. But in Hong Kong and Singapore's more relaxed regulatory environment, mini-bonds found willing sellers in the form of local banks and eager buyers among their customers.

Apparently, NLP techniques were deployed by Lehman Brothers, the top American investment banker, to make billions of dollars from the pools of easy meat or the less NLP conscious from Singapore and Hong Kong, outside the jurisdiction of the United States of America. NLP Yoga can protect you from people or institutions who are deliberately using the NLP operating manual to benefit themselves (offshore) un-ecologically at the expense of social stability and the welfare of your money by hacking and hijacking your unconscious operating manual. The fundamentals of analysis that we used to reveal the NLP packaged pseudo-bonds or pseudo-credit-linked notes is learned from Srimad Bhagavatam, a supplementary and compatible study along with the Gita, which does not require a prerequisite understanding in investment or finance.

Because we are ignorant of the subtle laws of nature (of the product nature), our endeavors for happiness in this world often only add to our distress.

> *lokah svayam shreyasi nashta-drishtir*
> *yo 'rthan samiheta nikama-kamah*
> *anyonya-vairah sukha-lesha-hetor*
> *ananta-duhkham cha na veda mudhah*

"Due to ignorance, the materialistic persons do not know anything about their real self-interest, the auspicious path in life. They are simply bound to material enjoyment by lusty desires, and all our plans are made for this purpose. For temporary sense gratification, such persons create a society of envy, and due to this mentality, they plunge into the ocean of suffering. Such a foolish person does not even know about this."

—*Srimad-Bhagavatam* 5.5.16

This is the description of the material world. *Anyonya-vairah:* Everyone is simply envious of one another. This is the material world: I am envious of you; you are envious of me. You can extend this principle to family, society, community, and nation, but the basic principle is envy, nothing else.

A verse in the beginning of the *Srimad-Bhagavatam* (1.1.2) describes who is fit to accept the spiritual principles of the *Bhagavatam*: dharmah projjhita-kaitavo 'tra paramo *nirmatsaraṇam*. The *Bhagavatam* is meant for persons who are no longer envious. Those who are envious have no entrance into the principles of *Srimad-Bhagavatam*.

The whole world is based on the principle of envy, *anyonya-vairah* . And what is the result of this envy? *Sukha-lesha-hetu*: temporary happiness.

PURPORT

The word *naṣṭa-dṛṣṭiḥ,* meaning "one who has no eyes to see the future," is very significant in this verse. (Product) Life goes on from one body to another, and the activities performed in this (product) life are enjoyed or suffered in the next life (after accumulator/minibonds scandal outburst), if not later in this life. One who is unintelligent, who has no eyes to see the future, simply creates enmity and fights with others for a sense of gratification. As a result, we suffer in the next life, but due to being like the blind, we continue to act in such a way that we suffer unlimitedly. Such persons are *mūḍha*, those who simply waste their time and do not understand the Lord's devotional service. As stated in *Bhagavad-gītā* (7.25):

> *nāhaṁ prakāśaḥ sarvasya*
> *yogamāyā-samāvṛtaḥ*
> *mūḍho 'yaṁ nābhijānāti*
> *loko mām ajam avyayam*

"I am never manifest to the foolish and unintelligent. For them I am covered by My eternal creative potency [*yogamāyā*]; and so the deluded world knows Me not, who am unborn and infallible."

In the *Kaṭha Upaniṣad* it is also said: *avidyāyām antare vartamānāḥ svayaṁ dhīrāḥ paṇḍitaṁmanyamānāḥ.* Ignorant people still go to other blind men for leadership. As a result, both are subjected to miserable conditions. The blind lead the blind into the ditch.

Now, you are gaining more seriousness and knowledge while reading this book. You will become more practical and pragmatic supported with values, street-smartness and excellent consciousness of sub-consciousness. Please follow each language that NLP Yoga programmed in this book. The language programmed in this book prepares your neurons to act in the bona fide way and for your maximum benefit, both in the material and spiritual domains.

So what is NLP? What is Yoga? Are NLP adherents the same as NLP Yoga? These will be outlined and explained throughout the book. Follow each word in this book diligently so that you won't miss any important points toward creating excellence or allow others to hijack your operating manual.

ARE YOU READY FOR THE MAIN COURSE?

Cruel history keeps repeating itself. There will be another bigger lesson to be learned which supersedes the I-kill-you-later or minibonds. To get liberated from this curse of law of nature, you need to be at full alert when studying the present based on recent history and first history/experience or even past life (lives). At present means if you want to achieve the state of a rich personality, you must <u>act</u> out a rich personality <u>now</u>. If you want to achieve the state of happiness, you must <u>act</u> happily <u>now</u>. It is better and easier to achieve the desired state by replacing the pain that you have previously collected/accumulated within your subconscious mind by learning NLP Yoga. However, never apply this "at present' strategy for your pain or negative emotion. "At present" is a two-edged sword. You can eternalize your pain or negative emotion too if you use it wrongly. Make sure you practice this together with other NLP Yogins when you first begin.

By observing the successful factors of a few contemporary international movements/leaderships, NLP Yoga resembles, strengthens and focuses toward driving desired results of NLP Yoga practitioners. Please note that NLP Yoga is not a study which digs into the negativity. NLP Yoga is not a blind faith and NLP Yoga does not study blind faith. NLP Yoga does not believe matters come from a void and enter into void. The existence of any matter has its own reasons. Just like you are attracted to this book. You are blessed, you are full of talents and you are being authenticated to your tastes. NLP Yoga comprehends the ancient wisdom with empowering language and makes it applicable for creating excellence in your personality for all aspects of your life.

From the few international movement examples later on, you will see that the reality you are living in is far bigger than you could tag with your own meanings/reasons. Let NLP Yoga empower you to create excellence in your personality. If you are looking forward to enacting transformation and improvement by solving problems at the root cause level, this is a must-read book for you whether you have lack of wealth, lack of motivation, lack of leadership, lack of acuity, lack of health, lack of love, lack of time, lack of confidence, lack of lightness, lack of humor, lack of formal education, lack of charisma, lack of liberalization, lack of conception, lack of mercy, lack of influence, etc.

THE AMWAY MOVEMENT

The first dish of your main course is the Amway Movement. **Amway** (short for The American Way) is an American company that uses a multi-level marketing model to sell a variety of products (from home care, personal care, jewelry, electronics, purifiers to insurance,etc). Based in Ada, Michigan, the company and family of companies under Alticor reported sales of $9.5 billion for 2015, the second consecutive year of decline for the company. Amway conducts business through a number of affiliated companies in more than a hundred countries and territories around the world. Amway was ranked No.26 among the largest private companies in the United States by *Forbes* in 2012. Amway has been subject to investigation as a pyramid scheme.

International expansion Amway expanded overseas to Australia in 1971, to Europe in 1973, to parts of Asia in 1974, to Japan in 1979, to Latin America in 1985, to Thailand in 1987, to China in 1995, to Africa in 1997, to India and Scandinavia in 1998, to Ukraine in 2003, to Russia in 2005, and to Vietnam in 2008. According to the Amway website, as of 2011 the company operates in over 100 countries and territories, organized into regional markets: the Americas, Europe, greater China, Japan and Korea, and South East Asia/Australia. The top ten markets for Amway in 2015 were China, South Korea, United States, Japan, Thailand, Russia, Taiwan, Malaysia, India and Ukraine.

In 2008, Alticor announced that two-thirds of the company's 58 markets reported sales increases, including strong growth in the China, Russia, Ukraine and India markets.

AMWAY CHINA

Amway grew quickly in China from its market launch in 1995. In 1998, after abuses of illegal pyramid schemes led to riots, the Chinese government enacted a ban on all direct selling companies, including Amway. After the negotiations, some companies like Amway, Avon, and Mary Kay continued to operate through a network of retail stores promoted by an independent sales force. China introduced new direct selling laws in December 2005, and in December 2006 Amway was one of the first companies to receive a license to resume direct sales. However, the law forbids teachers, doctors, and civil servants from becoming direct sales agents for the company and, unlike in the United States, salespeople in China are ineligible to receive commissions from sales made by the distributors they recruit.

In 2006, Amway China had reported 180,000 sales representatives, 140 stores, and $2 billion in annual sales. In 2007 Amway Greater China and South-east Asia Chief Executive Eva Cheng was ranked No.88 by *Forbes* magazine in its list of the World's

Most Powerful Women. In 2008, China was Amway's largest market, reporting 28% growth and sales of ¥17 billion (US$2.5 billion). According to a report in Bloomberg Business Week in April 2010, Amway had 237 retail shops in China, 160,000 direct sales agents, and $3 billion in revenue.

FTC INVESTIGATION ON AMWAY

Robert Carroll, of the *Skeptic's Dictionary*, has described Amway as a "legal pyramid scheme," and has said that the quasi-religious devotion of its affiliates is used by the company to conceal poor performance rates by distributors.

In a 1979 ruling, the Federal Trade Commission found that Amway does not fit the definition of a pyramid scheme because (a) distributors were not paid to recruit people, (b) it did not require distributors to buy a large stock of unmoving inventory, (c) distributors were required to maintain retail sales (at least 10 per month), and (d) the company and all distributors were required to accept returns of excess inventory from down-level distributors.

The FTC did, however, find Amway "guilty of price-fixing and making exaggerated income claims." The company was ordered to stop retail price fixing and allocating customers among distributors and was prohibited from misrepresenting the amount of profit, earnings or sales its distributors are likely to achieve with the business. Amway was ordered to accompany any such statements with the actual averages per distributor, pointing out that more than half of the distributors do not make any money, with the average distributor making less than $100 per month. The order was violated with a 1986 ad campaign, resulting in a $100,000 fine.

AMWAY CULTISM

Some Amway distributor groups have been accused of using "cult-like" tactics to attract new distributors and keep them involved and committed. Allegations include resemblance to a Big Brother organization with paranoid attitude to insiders critical of the organization, seminars and rallies resembling religious revival meetings and enormous involvement of distributors despite minimal incomes. An examination of the 1979–1980 tax records in the state of Wisconsin showed that the direct distributors reported a net loss of $918 on average.

NLP YOGA'S OBSERVATIONS

Any NLP Yogin will never be satisfied with fed information from open sources. As a normal practice, NLP Yogin will dig down to look for greater details. According to its 2015 annual report published at Bursa Malaysia, http://www.bursamalaysia.com/market/listed-companies/company-announcements/5062809, Amway (Malaysia) Holdings Berhad, 51.7% owned by GDA B.V. http://www.bloomberg.com/Research/stocks/private/snapshot.asp?privcapId=28387825 ,reported MYR1.0199 Billion Sales Revenue. More than three quarters of 2015 MYR (The Malaysian Ringgit) was traded above the four mark to USD1.00. Translating this MYR1.0199 into USD at four mark would mean USD254,975,000. GDA B.V., the Amway private holding company's 51.7% shares in Amway (Malaysia) Holdings Berhad means sales revenues of less than USD132 million contribution to the Amway global sales revenue during the period (some may suggest better use cost of goods sold by the AMWAY USA to AMWAY Malaysia as a basis of calculation. It is up to you, as we are not going into the accounting with precision). Malaysia as the top 8th market of AMWAY contributed less than 1.4% of the global sales revenue in 2015. Obviously and certainly, the top-heavy distribution of performance of global sale revenue of Amway deserves more digging down for details. According to http://www.thetruthaboutamway.com/amway-sales-top-10-countries-2012/, more truths are revealed in 2012:

AMWAY SALES – TOP 10 COUNTRIES 2012

Country	Sales (USD$m)	Growth
China	$4,385	+1%
Japan	$1,185	+2%
Korea	$885	+2%
United States	$861	+5%
Russia	$629	+19%
Thailand	$568	+10%
India	$493	+7%
Taiwan	$340	+8%
Malaysia	$263	+8%
Ukraine	$150	+7%

source: Amway Europe Leadership Training Seminar 2013

Summing up the total sales of the above table yields USD9,757M. As a USA based company, USA only accounted for less than 9% for the global sales revenue and China's contribution was almost 45%. Amway USA was founded in 1959. Amway China started in 1995, was banned in 1998 and reobtained its business license to operate near the end of 2006. What made Amway China overtake Amway USA by five times in 2012? Amway China must have exceeded Amway USA years before 2012. Again, NLP Yoga's objective is not to look for precision in facts and figures but the root cause.

Guess what? GDP or GDP per capita? Emerging? Growing? Consumer behavior? Quality of products? Population? Market size? All are possible. However, when you are given financial statements or presentation materials, the best answers are always off the financial statement or presentation material. It is more important, that is, because of the linguistic medium, the language that is widely used in China which is (Simplified) Putonghua/Mandarin. Simplified Putonghua (contains less strokes and can be easier, efficient and effective to remember/recognize in written form by either native, new or alien learners) is a very **NLP** effective and friendly language, especially in business. China has more than 160 dialects and Putonghua (because it is simplified/reinvented by a group of professional linguists) is overwhelming and flooding the entire Mainland China since its nationwide introduction in the 1950s. Now switch to the world second largest population, India. India's population is not lagging too far behind China. However, the caste system and diverse languages available in different localities in India are causing ineffectiveness for the linguistic flow effectively throughout the country. There are twenty-two major languages in India, written in thirteen different scripts, with over 720 dialects. The official Indian languages are Hindi (with approximately 420 million speakers) and English, which is also widely spoken. In addition, several states in India have their own official languages, which are usually only spoken in particular areas. Among them are *Bengali* (83 million speakers), *Telugu* (spoken by 74 million people) and *Marathi* (72 million speakers).

Language and words used are very important according to NLP and the Gita, as you will see later. The words that a user/leader use will determine a team's outcome. NLP Yoga will elaborate at greater length regarding this in a later part of the book.

THE NEURO-LINGUISTIC PROGRAMMING MOVEMENT

Interesting, very interesting. We are now about to enter into the neuro-linguistic programming movement. This information on the neuro-linguistic programming movement is important feedback to the further development of NLP and thus gives birth to NLP Yoga. **Neuro-linguistic programming** (**NLP**) is the study of how you think, speak verbally and behave with body language. Now if you are looking to study "How you are getting what you are getting," NLP is a good place to begin. As a wise man once said **"To change your outcome it is important that you change your thinking."** Easier said than done. It is a process of understanding our own selves by observing and understanding the world around us (or vice versa), with a new set of very successful methodologies, tools and techniques, evolved in the world of **NLP** by experts.

Neuro-linguistic programming (**NLP**) is an approach to communication, personal development, and psychotherapy created by Richard Bandler and John Grinder in California, United States during the 1970s. Grinder is an American linguist, author, management consultant, trainer and speaker. Bandler is an American author and trainer in the field of self-help. NLP has since been overwhelmingly discredited scientifically by people who are not familiar with NLP, but NLP continues to be marketed by some hypnotherapists and by some companies that organize seminars and workshops on management training for businesses.

Bandler and Grinder claim there is a connection between neurological processes (*neuro-*), language (*linguistic*) and behavioral patterns learned through experience (*programming*), and that these can be changed to achieve specific goals in life. Bandler and Grinder also claim that NLP methodology can "model" the skills of exceptional people, allowing anyone to acquire those skills. They claim as well that, often in a single session, NLP can treat problems such as phobias, depression, tic disorders, psychosomatic illnesses, near-sightedness, allergy, common cold, and learning disorders.

There is no scientific evidence supporting the claims made by NLP advocates and it has been discredited as a pseudoscience by experts who are not familiar with NLP. Scientific reviews state that NLP is based on outdated metaphors of how the brain works that are inconsistent with current neurological theory and contain numerous factual errors. Reviews by these people also found that all of the supportive research on NLP contained significant methodological flaws and that there were three times as many studies of a much higher quality that failed to reproduce the "extraordinary claims" made by Bandler, Grinder, and other NLP practitioners. Even so, NLP has been adopted by some hypnotherapists and also by companies that run seminars marketed as leadership training to businesses and government agencies.

EARLY DEVELOPMENT OF NLP

According to Bandler and Grinder, NLP comprises a methodology termed *modeling*, plus a set of techniques that they derived from its initial applications. Of such methods that are considered fundamental, they derived many from the work of Virginia Satir, Milton Erickson and Fritz Perls.

Bandler and Grinder also drew upon the theories of Gregory Bateson, Alfred Korzybski and Noam Chomsky (particularly transformational grammar), as well as ideas and techniques from Carlos Castaneda.

Bandler and Grinder claim that their methodology can codify the structure inherent to the therapeutic "magic" as performed in therapy by Perls, Satir and Erickson, and indeed inherent to any complex human activity, and then from that codification, the structure and its activity can be learned by others. Their book published in 1975, *The Structure of Magic I: A Book about Language and Therapy*, is intended to be a codification of the therapeutic techniques of Perls and Satir.

Bandler and Grinder say that they used their own process of *modeling* to model Virginia Satir so they could produce what they termed the *Meta-Model*, a model for gathering information and challenging a client's language and underlying thinking. They claim that by challenging linguistic distortions, specifying generalizations, and recovering deleted information in the client's statements, the transformational grammar concepts of *surface structure* yield a more complete representation of the underlying *deep structure* and therefore have therapeutic benefit. Also derived from Satir were *anchoring*, *future pacing* and *representational systems*.

In contrast, the *Milton-Model*—a model of the purportedly hypnotic language of Milton Erickson—was described by Bandler and Grinder as "artfully vague" and metaphoric. The Milton-Model is used in combination with the Meta-Model as a softener, to induce a "trance" and to deliver indirect therapeutic suggestion.

However, adjunct lecturer in linguistics, Karen Stollznow, describes Bandler's and Grinder's reference to such experts as namedropping. Other than Satir, the people they cite as influences did not collaborate with Bandler or Grinder. Chomsky himself has no association with NLP whatsoever; his original work was intended as theory, not therapy. Stollznow writes, "[o]ther than borrowing terminology, NLP does not bear authentic resemblance to any of Chomsky's theories or philosophies – linguistic, cognitive or political."

According to André Muller Weitzenhoffer, a researcher in the field of hypnosis, "the major weakness of Bandler and Grinder's linguistic analysis is that so much of it is built upon untested hypotheses and is supported by totally inadequate data." Weitzenhoffer adds that Bandler and Grinder misuse formal logic and mathematics,[1] redefine or misunderstand terms from the linguistics lexicon (*e.g.*, nominalization), create a scientific façade by needlessly complicating Ericksonian concepts with unfounded claims, make factual errors, and disregard or confuse concepts central to the Ericksonian approach.

More recently (circa 1997), Bandler has claimed, "NLP is based on finding out what works and formalizing it. In order to formalize patterns, I utilized everything from linguistics to holography...The models that constitute NLP are all formal models based on mathematical, logical principles such as predicate calculus and the mathematical equations underlying holography."[1] However, there is no mention of the mathematics of holography nor of holography in general in McClendon's, Spitzer's, or Grinder's account of the development of NLP.

On the matter of the development of NLP, Grinder recollects:

My memories about what we thought at the time of discovery (with respect to the classic code we developed – that is, the years 1973 through 1978) are that we were quite explicit that we were out to overthrow a paradigm and that, for example, I, for one, found it very useful to plan this campaign using in part as a guide the excellent work of Thomas Kuhn (*The Structure of Scientific Revolutions*) in which he detailed some of the conditions which historically have been obtained in the midst of paradigm shifts. For example, I believe it was very useful that neither one of us were qualified in the field we first went after – psychology and, in particular, its therapeutic application; this being one of the conditions which Kuhn identified in his historical study of paradigm shifts.

The philosopher, Robert Todd Carroll, responded that Grinder has not understood Kuhn's text on the history and philosophy of science, *The Structure of Scientific Revolutions*. Carroll replies: (a) individual scientists never have nor are they ever able to create *paradigm shifts* volitionally and Kuhn does not suggest otherwise; (b) Kuhn's text does not contain the idea that being unqualified in a field of science is a prerequisite to producing a result that necessitates a *paradigm shift* in that field and (c) *The Structure of Scientific Revolutions* is foremost a work of *history* and not an instructive text on *creating* paradigm shifts and such a text is not possible—extraordinary discovery is not a formulaic procedure. Carroll explains that a *paradigm shift* is not a planned activity, rather it is an outcome of scientific effort within the current (dominant) paradigm that produces data that can't be adequately accounted for within the current paradigm—hence a *paradigm shift*, i.e. the adoption of a new paradigm.

In developing NLP, Bandler and Grinder were not responding to a paradigmatic crisis in psychology nor did they produce any data that caused a paradigmatic crisis in psychology. There is no sense in which Bandler and Grinder caused or participated in a paradigm shift. What did Grinder and Bandler do that makes it impossible to continue doing psychology…without accepting their ideas? "Nothing," argues Carroll.

COMMERCIALIZATION OF NLP AND EVALUATION

By the late 1970s, the human potential movement had developed into an industry and provided a market for some NLP ideas. At the center of this growth was the Esalen Institute

THE NEURO-LINGUISTIC PROGRAMMING MOVEMENT

at Big Sur, California. Perls had led numerous Gestalt therapy seminars at Esalen. Satir was an early leader and Bateson was a guest teacher. Bandler and Grinder claimed that in addition to being a therapeutic method, NLP was also a study of communication and began marketing it as a business tool, claiming that, "if any human being can do anything, so can you."

After 150 students paid $1,000 each for a ten-day workshop in Santa Cruz, California, Bandler and Grinder gave up academic writing and produced popular books from seminar transcripts, such as *Frogs into Princes,* which sold more than 270,000 copies. According to court documents relating to an intellectual property dispute between Bandler and Grinder, Bandler made more than $800,000 in 1980 from workshop and book sales. Taking inflation into account, the value of $800,000 in 1980 was worth $2.47 Million in 2016. (http://www.saving.org/inflation/inflation.php?amount=80,000&year=1980)

A community of psychotherapists and students began to form around Bandler and Grinder's initial works, leading to the growth and spread of NLP as a theory and practice. For example, Tony Robbins trained with Grinder and utilized a few ideas from NLP as part of his own self-help and motivational speaking programs. Bandler led several unsuccessful efforts to exclude other parties from using NLP. Meanwhile, the rising number of practitioners and theorists led NLP to become even less uniform than it was at its foundation. Prior to the decline of NLP, scientific researchers began testing its theoretical underpinnings empirically, with research indicating a lack of empirical support for NLP's essential theories. The 1990s were characterized by fewer scientific studies evaluating the methods of NLP than during the previous decade. Tomasz Witkowski attributes this to a declining interest in the debate as a result of a lack of empirical support for NLP from its proponents.

Main components and core concepts of NLP

NLP can be understood in terms of three broad components and the central concepts pertaining to those:

- *Subjectivity.* According to Bandler and Grinder:

  - We experience the world subjectively; thus we create subjective representations of our experience. These subjective representations of experience are constituted in terms of five senses and language. That is to say our subjective conscious experience is in terms of the traditional senses of vision, audition, tactition, olfaction and gustation such that when we—for example—rehearse an activity "in our heads," recall an event or anticipate the future, we will "see" images, "hear" sounds, "taste" flavors, "feel" tactile sensations, "smell" odors and think in some (natural) language. Furthermore it is claimed that these subjective representations of experience have a discernible structure, a pattern. It is in this sense that NLP is sometimes defined as *the study of the structure of subjective experience*.

- Behavior can be described and understood in terms of these sense-based subjective representations. Behavior is broadly conceived to include verbal and non-verbal communication, incompetent, maladaptive or "pathological" behavior as well as effective or skillful behavior.

- Behavior (in self and others) can be modified by manipulating these sense-based subjective representations.

- **Consciousness.** NLP is predicated on the notion that consciousness is bifurcated into a conscious component and an unconscious component. Those subjective representations that occur outside of an individual's awareness comprise what is referred to as the "unconscious mind."

- **Learning.** NLP utilizes an imitative method of learning—termed *modeling*—that is claimed to be able to codify and reproduce an exemplar's expertise in any domain of activity. An important part of the codification process is a description of the sequence of the sensory/linguistic representations of the subjective experience of the exemplar during execution of the expertise.

Techniques or set of practices

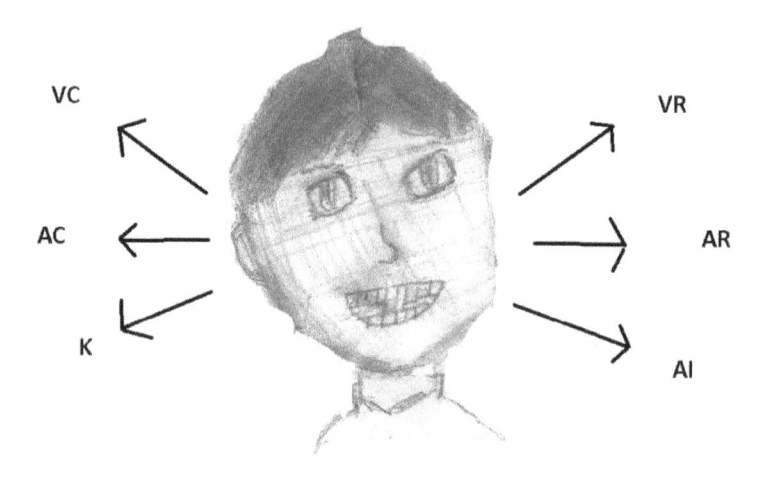

An "eye accessing cue chart" as it appears in an example in Bandler & Grinder's Frogs into Princes (1979). The six directions represent "visual construct," "visual recall," "auditory construct," "auditory recall." "kinesthetic" and "auditory internal dialogue."

According to one study by Steinbach, a classic interaction in NLP can be understood in terms of several major stages including establishing rapport, gleaning information about a problematic mental state and desired goals, using specific tools and techniques to make interventions, and integrating proposed changes into the client's life. The entire process is guided by the non-verbal responses of the client. The first is the act of establishing and maintaining rapport between the practitioner and the client which is achieved through pacing and leading the verbal (*e.g.*, sensory predicates and keywords) and non-verbal behavior (*e.g.*, matching and mirroring non-verbal behavior, or responding to eye movements) of the client.

THE NEURO-LINGUISTIC PROGRAMMING MOVEMENT

Once rapport is established, the practitioner may gather information (*e.g.*, using the meta-model questions) about the client's present state as well as help the client define a desired state or goal for the interaction. The practitioner pays particular attention to the verbal and non-verbal responses as the client defines the present state and desired state and any "resources" that may be required to bridge the gap. The client is typically encouraged to consider the consequences of the desired outcome, and how they may affect his or her personal or professional life and relationships, taking into account any positive intentions of any problems that may arise (i.e. ecological check). Fourth, the practitioner assists the client in achieving the desired outcomes by using certain tools and techniques to change internal representations and responses to stimuli in the world. Finally, the changes are "future paced" by helping the client to mentally rehearse and integrate the changes into his or her life. For example, the client may be asked to "step into the future" and represent (mentally see, hear and feel) what it is like having already achieved the outcome.

According to Stollznow (2010), "NLP also involves fringe discourse analysis and "practical" guidelines for "improved" communication. For example, one text asserts "when you adopt the 'but' word, people will remember what you said afterwards. With the 'and' word, people remember what you said before and after."

Applications

Alternative medicine

In the earlier days, some NLP has been promoted with claims it can be used to treat a variety of diseases including Parkinson's disease, HIV/AIDS and cancer. Such claims have no supporting medical evidence. People who use NLP only as a form of treatment risk serious adverse health consequences as it can delay the provision of effective medical care.

Psychotherapeutic

Early books about NLP had a psychotherapeutic focus, given that the early models were psychotherapists. As an approach to psychotherapy, NLP shares similar core assumptions and foundations in common with some contemporary brief and systemic practices, such as solution-focused brief therapy. NLP has also been acknowledged as having influenced these practices with its reframing techniques which seeks to achieve behavioral change by shifting its *context* or *meaning*, for example, by finding the positive connotation of a thought or behavior.

The two main therapeutic uses of NLP are: (1) as an adjunct by therapists practicing in other therapeutic disciplines; (2) as a specific therapy called neurolinguistics psychotherapy which is recognized by the United Kingdom Council for Psychotherapy with accreditation governed at first by the Association for Neuro-Linguistic Programming and more recently by its daughter organization the Neuro Linguistic Psychotherapy and

Counseling Association. Neither neuro-linguistic programming nor neuro-linguistic psychotherapy are NICE-approved.

According to Stollznow (2010) "Bandler and Grinder's infamous *Frogs into Princes* and their other books boast that NLP is a cure-all that treats a broad range of physical and mental conditions and learning difficulties, including epilepsy, myopia and dyslexia. With its promises to cure schizophrenia, depression and post-traumatic stress disorder, and its dismissal of psychiatric illnesses as psychosomatic, NLP shares similarities with Scientology and the Citizens Commission on Human Rights (CCHR)." A systematic review of experimental studies by Sturt *et al* (2012) concluded that "there is little evidence that NLP interventions improve health-related outcomes." In his review of NLP, Stephen Briers writes, "NLP is not really a cohesive therapy but a ragbag of different techniques without a particularly clear theoretical basis [and its] evidence base is virtually non-existent." Eisner writes, "NLP appears to be a superficial and gimmicky approach to dealing with mental health problems. Unfortunately, NLP appears to be the first in a long line of mass marketing seminars that purport to virtually cure any mental disorder...it appears that NLP has no empirical or scientific support as to the underlying tenets of its theory or clinical effectiveness. What remains is a mass-marketed serving of psychopablum."

André Muller Weitzenhoffer—a friend and peer of Milton Erickson—wrote, "Has NLP really abstracted and explicated the essence of successful therapy and provided everyone with the means to be another Whittaker, Virginia Satir, or

Erickson?...[NLP's] failure to do this is evident because today there is no multitude of their equals, not even another Whittaker, Virginia Satir, or Erickson. Ten years should have been sufficient time for this to happen. In this light, I cannot take NLP seriously...[NLP's] contributions to our understanding and use of Ericksonian techniques are equally dubious. *Patterns I* and *II* are poorly written works that were an overambitious, pretentious effort to reduce hypnotism to a magic of words."

Clinical psychologist Stephen Briers questions the value of the NLP maxim—a *presupposition* in NLP jargon—"there is no failure, only feedback." Briers argues that the denial of the existence of failure diminishes its instructive value. He offers experiences of Walt Disney, Isaac Newton and J.K. Rowling as three examples of unambiguous acknowledged personal failure that served as an impetus to great success. According to Briers, it was "the crash-and-burn type of failure, not the sanitized NLP Failure Lite, i.e. the failure-that-isn't really-failure sort of failure" that propelled these individuals to success. Briers contends that adherence to the maxim leads to self-deprecation. According to Briers, personal endeavor is a product of invested values and aspirations and the dismissal of personally significant failure as mere feedback effectively denigrates what one values. Briers writes, "Sometimes we need to accept and mourn the death of our dreams, not just casually dismiss them as inconsequential. NLP's reframe casts us into the role of a widower avoiding the pain of grief by leap-frogging into a rebound relationship with a younger woman, never pausing to say a proper goodbye to his dead wife." Briers also contends that the NLP maxim is narcissistic, self-centered and divorced from notions of moral responsibility.

Other uses

Although the original core techniques of NLP were therapeutic in orientation their genericity enabled them to be applied to other fields. These applications include persuasion,[1] sales, negotiation, management training, sports, teaching, coaching, team building, and public speaking.

Scientific criticism

In the early 1980s, NLP was advertised as an important advance in psychotherapy and counseling, and attracted some interest in counseling research and clinical psychology. However, as controlled trials failed to show any benefit from NLP and its advocates made increasingly dubious claims, scientific interest in NLP faded. Numerous literature reviews and meta-analyses have failed to show evidence for NLP's assumptions or effectiveness as a therapeutic method.[90] While some NLP practitioners have argued that the lack of empirical support is due to insufficient research testing NLP, the consensus scientific opinion is that NLP is pseudoscience and that attempts to dismiss the research findings based on these arguments "[constitute]s an admission that NLP does not have an evidence base and that NLP practitioners are seeking a post-hoc credibility." Surveys in the academic community have shown NLP to be widely discredited among scientists. Among the reasons for considering NLP a pseudoscience are that evidence in favor of it is limited to anecdotes and personal testimony, that it is not informed by scientific understanding of neuroscience and linguistics, and that the name "neuro-linguistic programming" uses jargon words to impress readers and obfuscate ideas, whereas NLP itself does not relate any phenomena to neural structures and has nothing in common with linguistics or programming. In fact, in education, NLP has been used as a key example of pseudoscience.

As a quasi-religion

Sociologists and anthropologists—among others—have categorized NLP as a quasi-religion belonging to the New Age and/or human potential movements. Medical anthropologist Jean M. Langford categorizes NLP as a form of folk magic; that is to say, a practice with symbolic efficacy—as opposed to physical efficacy—that is able to effect change through nonspecific effects (*e.g.*, placebo effect). To Langford, NLP is akin to a syncretic folk religion "that attempts to wed the magic of folk practice to the science of professional medicine." Bandler and Grinder were (and continue to be) influenced by the shamanism described in the books of Carlos Castaneda. Several ideas and techniques have been borrowed from Castaneda and incorporated into NLP including so-called *double induction* and the notion of "stopping the world" which is central to NLP modeling. Tye (1994) characterizes NLP as a type of "psycho shamanism." Fanthorpe and Fanthorpe (2008) see a similarity between the mimetic procedure and intent of NLP modeling and aspects of ritual in some syncretic religions. Hunt (2003) draws a comparison between the concern with lineage from an NLP guru—which is evident among some

NLP proponents—and the concern with guru lineage in some Eastern religions.

In Aupers and Houtman (2010) Bovbjerg identifies NLP as a New Age "psycho-religion" and uses NLP as a case-study to demonstrate the thesis that the New Age psycho-religions such as NLP are predicated on an intrinsically religious idea, namely concern with a transcendent "other." In the world's monotheistic faiths, argues Bovbjerg, the purpose of religious practice is communion and fellowship with a transcendent 'other,' i.e. a God. With the New Age psycho-religions, argues Bovbjerg, this orientation toward a transcendent 'other' persists but the *other* has become "the other in ourselves," the so-called *unconscious*: "[t]he individual's inner life becomes the intangible focus of [psycho-]religious practices and the subconscious becomes a constituent part of modern individuals' understanding of the Self." Bovbjerg adds, "[C]ourses in personal development would make no sense without an unconscious that contains hidden resources and hidden knowledge of the self." Thus psycho-religious practice revolves around ideas of the conscious and unconscious self and communicating with and accessing the hidden resources of the unconscious self—the transcendent *other*. According to Bovbjerg the notion that we have an unconscious self underlies many NLP techniques either explicitly or implicitly. Bovbjerg argues, "[t]hrough particular practices, the [NLP practitioner*qua*] psycho-religious practitioner expects to achieve self-perfection in a never-ending transformation of the self."

Bovbjerg's secular critique of NLP is echoed in the conservative Christian perspective of the New Age as represented by Jeremiah (1995) who argues that, "[t]he 'transformation' recommended by the founders and leaders of these business seminars [such as NLP] has spiritual implications that a non-Christian or new believer may not recognize. The belief that human beings can change themselves by calling upon the power (or god) within or their own infinite human potential is a contradiction of the Christian view. The Bible says mankind is a sinner and is saved by God's grace alone."

SOME FAMOUS PEOPLE WHO USED NLP TO CREATE EXCELLENCE

The feedback on NLP on the previous pages is quite one-sided. Perhaps the feedback was provided by non-believers of NLP. You may even think that this book should say everything good about NLP. What is the motive or intention that this book brings out about the NLP movement and the feedback that people are providing to NLP? Let's move from academic argument to look at the successful side of the real story. Like Gautama Buddha said, "there were many Buddhas before me, there are many Buddhas who co-exist with me at present and there will be many more Buddhas after me, the philosophy of NLP existed long before Bandler and Grinder published their works in the 1970s.

Below are some of the famous people who used NLP (hypnosis is a major part of NLP) to create excellence:

> Albert Einstein. Other famous people in history known to have used hypnosis are Thomas Edison (inventor), Henry Ford (car manufacturer), Sir Winston Churchill and Jackie Kennedy

Jimmy Carr. Other famous people reported to use and love NLP are Heston Blumental, Lily Allen, Gerri Halliwell and Sophie Dahl.

Anthony Robbins says of NLP 'I built my sales career from zero to become the world's best motivator using NLP.'

Oprah Winfrey says of NLP 'NLP helps me to manage audiences and motivate them. It is amazing.'

Warren Buffett and Andre Agassi are understood to have used NLP to achieve inspirational results.

Pharrell Williams talks about his use of and love for NLP in a Psychology Today article: 'I am a huge NLP person. I love NLP.'

Cheryl Fernandez-Versini (Cole) reportedly used NLP to help her build back her confidence after her marriage breakdown and being ditched from X Factor. Once you have learned to use tools, they are skills for life. You can use them to help you through difficult periods and to rebuild yourself when tough things happen (like they do to everyone).

Russell Brand openly declares NLP as a lifesaver when he used it to get over his self-destructive patterns.

It is not the purpose of this book to provide a full and exhaustive list of famous NLP practitioners. To sum up here, John F.

Kennedy, Martin Luther King, Robert Kennedy, Bill Clinton, Barack Obama and Tony Blair all have been trained in NLP. Please note that the above feedback is made by some very high profile personalities.

We live in a world of duality like a two-sided coin. There are people who say it's a *head* and they are people arguing that it is a *tail*. If something is not *science*, we can accept it as an *art* or simply acknowledge it is not *science*. As long as it is useful and can be modeled. NLP Yogin do not spend unproductive time in heated discussion which runs into lengthy argument or unstoppable resentment.

BANDLER AND GRINDER FELL APART JUST BEFORE NLP BECAME MORE ACCEPTABLE AND LESS FLAWED.

By the end of 1980, the collaboration between Bandler and Grinder ended. On 25 September 1981, Bandler instituted a civil action against Grinder and his company, seeking injunctive relief and damages for Grinder's commercial activity in relation to NLP. On 29 October 1981, judgment was made in favor of Bandler. As part of a settlement agreement, Bandler granted to Grinder a limited 10-year license to conduct NLP seminars, offer certification in NLP and use the NLP name on the condition that royalties from the earnings of the seminars be paid to Bandler. In July 1996 and January 1997, Bandler instituted a further two civil actions against Grinder and his company, numerous other prominent figures in NLP and 200 further initially unnamed persons. Bandler alleged that Grinder had violated the terms of the settlement agreement reached in the initial case and he had suffered commercial damage as a result of the allegedly illegal commercial activities of the defendants. Bandler sought from *each* defendant damages no less than $10,000,000. In February 2000, the court found against Bandler, stating that "Bandler has misrepresented to the public through his licensing agreement and promotional materials, that he was the exclusive owner of all intellectual property rights associated with NLP, and maintained the exclusive authority to determine membership in and certification in the Society of NLP.

On this matter Stollznow (2010) comments, "[I]ronically, Bandler and Grinder feuded in the 1980s over trademark and theory disputes. Tellingly, none of their myriad of NLP models, pillars, and principles helped these founders to resolve their personal and professional conflicts.

In December 1997, Tony Clarkson instituted civil proceedings against Bandler to have Bandler's UK trademark of NLP revoked. The court found in favor of Clarkson; Bandler's trademark was subsequently revoked.

WIN-WIN SITUATION IS A STATE OF STABILITY AND PERMANENCE

"Annica, Anicca. Impermanence, Impermanence." Change is inherent in all phenomenal existence. There is nothing animate or inanimate, organic or inorganic that we can label as permanent, since even as we affix that label on something it would undergo metamorphosis. Realizing this central fact of life by direct experience within himself, the Buddha declared, "Whether a fully Enlightened One has arisen in the world or not, it still remains a firm condition, an immutable fact and fixed law that all formations are impermanent, subject to suffering, and devoid of substance." *Anicca* (impermanence), *dukkha* (suffering), and *anatta* (insubstantiality) are the three characteristics common to all sentient existence.

By the end of 2000, Bandler and Grinder entered a release where they agreed, among other things, that "they are the co-creators and co-founders of the technology of neuro-linguistic programming" and "mutually agree to refrain from disparaging each other's efforts, in any fashion, concerning their respective involvement in the field of Neuro-linguistic Programming.

As a consequence of these disputes and settlements, the names *NLP* and *Neuro-linguistic Programming* are not owned by any party and there is no restriction on any party offering NLP certification.

Lord Palmerston, 19th century UK prime minister and foreign secretary once said: "Nations have no permanent friends or allies, they only have permanent interests." No wonder statesmen in Parliament do not give a dime to people seeking self-enlightenment under the tree. To run a country requires more wisdom than self-enlightenment. Some world-renowned leaders (John F. Kennedy, Martin Luther King, Robert Kennedy, Bill Clinton, Barack Obama and Tony Blair) acquire techniques from NLP and some (Gandhi, Modi, Cameron, Obama, etc) acquire wisdom from the Gita.

THE FIRE WITHIN BHAGAVAD GITA

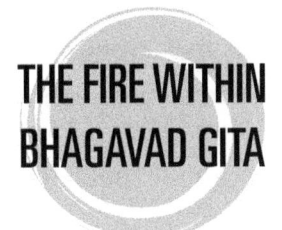

Bob Nelson once said, "You get the best effort from others not by lighting a fire beneath them, but by building a fire within." The Gita is such a book which builds fire within. Before even speaking about the Gita, we could not afford to leave out the true story of His Divine Grace A.C. Bhaktivedanta Swami Srila Prabhupada, the authoritative translator and author of 'Bhagavad Gita As It Is'. At the age of 70, he came to the streets of New York, USA during 1996, penniless and homeless. At his disappearance on 1977, he left with the below stunning results:

- He opened 108 Hare Krishna temples (Steve Jobs loved and walked the seven miles across town every Sunday night to get one good meal a week from the Hare Krishna temple near him) in six continents

- He circumnavigated the globe fourteen times sharing his message with millions

- He authorized over 70 books, including his famous bestseller, the Bhagavad Gita: As It is, which have sold billions of copies to date

- He inspired thousands of people to break free from all bad habits and lead a life of selfless service to humanity

How did he manage to do all that after age 70? This was his earlier life till 1966:

- From 1923-1953 he ran a small pharmaceutical shop to financially assist his guru's mission, but his shop was burglarized and ruined

- From 1944 to 1960, he ran a magazine, Back to Godhead, to spread the message of spiritual love, single-handedly writing, typing, proofreading, publishing and distributing. The magazine found few takers.

- From 1952 to 1954, he invested all his time, energy and finances to establish an organization, The League of Devotees, in India, but he was evicted by political intrigue

- During 1965, when aged 69, he decided to go to the USA alone and penniless to share his message. He had two heart attacks on the ship which almost killed Him on the oceans.

- During 1966, he tried to build a temple in USA with financial assistance from the patron from India, as a foreign exchange control regime, the Indian government refused to let the Indian financial assistance to flow out of the country

- During 1966, while he focused on sharing His message with young Americans, his first serious student went crazy due to drug overdose and attacked Him. He had to flee for his life.

He had encountered so many challenges, obstacles, tests, austerities and many more reversals before. Most people would have just given up at his age. But He was beyond all material success and failures. His indomitable spirit came from his living and working on the divine platform as he explained to a disheartened student in 1969: "So I don't think there is any cause of discouragement because we are working on a different platform."

The life story of the author of 'Bhagavad Gita: As It is' is such a book of motivation and leadership. Now let's turn toward the essence of the Gita and see how much NLP relates to the Gita, unconsciously or knowingly but latently.

FAST AND FURIOUS MOTIVATION

The Gita literally means Song of the Absolute. It is a conversation between Arjuna (as if conscious mind in modern speech) and Krishna (as if subconscious mind in modern speech), which took place around 3000 B.C. on a Kurukshetra battlefield which Arjuna needed to fight with his own people. Krishna represents the Supreme Being who appeared as charioteer to Arjuna. Arjuna represents an ordinary living being with prescribed social duty-warrior. Arjuna is also the best archer of his time and a great leader. The Gita is a discussion between two leaders (Krishna, the divine leader (subconscious mind leader), and Arjuna the material leader (conscious mind leader) about the right course of action and the basis for it during a fast and furious moment. There are two battlefields actually. One is the physical battlefield and another is Arjuna's internal battlefield. Just when the war was about to start, Arjuna was overcome with self-doubt about the righteousness of the war against his own kith and kin. He was distraught and struggled at the thought of having to fight with his friends and family, and others, such as his dear teacher. With this emotional breakdown he copped out, and Arjuna refused to fight. It was then, surrounded by enemies in the battlefield, that Krishna empowered Arjuna by explaining the necessity and inevitability of the war to Arjuna. Arjuna plays the role of the seeker in the Gita and Krishna dispenses the advice. With Krishna's powerful words, Arjuna felt motivated and without further hesitation during the crucial do-it-or-die time he turned his doubt into faith, led his warriors and fought and won in a powerful battle.

THE ROLE OF LEADERS

The role of leaders is explicitly outlined. In the Gita (3.21), it says, "Whatever course of action a superior man pursues, lesser persons will follow and the world will accept the standard he sets." The science and knowledge of leadership were taught and learned by leaders through disciplic succession (4.1, 4.2). In (1.46), we learn about how a negative emotional state of

Arjuna can result in refusal to perform socially prescribed duties/professions/jobs. The atmosphere at the battlefield was frenzied and tense. However the tone of voice of Krishna was calm, His words were precisely reasoned and His demeanor was unflappably composed while talking to Arjuna. As a result, Arjuna was intellectually illumined, spiritually strengthened, emotionally enlivened and understood his purpose of life-facing and learning from life instead of hiding and allowing painful emotion to overwhelm his learning.

THE LAW OF NATURE AND HOW TO BE GUIDED

The law of nature is explained in the Gita (9.10) "It is through Me alone that *prakriti* brings the moving and non-moving beings into existence, for I am the Controller. This is the designated cause by means of which the world proceeds on its course." In the Gita (18.61) we are told that the guidance and knowledge of the law of nature are not remote externally but present right in our hearts. Thus, we must tune our consciousness to the frequency of law of nature and listen to the inner voice rather than following negative self talk or the fancies of a ventriloquist. Leaders are the ones who face adversities with maturity because leaders need to overcome inhibitions with aspirations for inner victory before they can lead to fight the external war.

WISDOM OF SELF REALIZATION

In the Gita (9.2), absolute truth is the purest king of knowledge, secret of all secrets. It gives direct perception of the self by realization. It is everlasting and joyful when performed. Just like you won't need an engineering degree and special training to know whether a two –door Porsche can plough a padi field joyfully.

DISASSOCIATION AND STAYING ABOVE THE SUBJECT MATTER

The famous and effective disassociation technique used by NLP was originated from the Gita. It is a strategy to allow us to stay concerned yet not personally involved and disturbed by external events. For example, if we are standing at the foot of a volcano, we feel threatened but if we were in an aircraft flying above the volcano, then the feeling of being threatened is not so immediate. The volcano is still there. However your perception has changed because your perspective and the position from where you look at the subject matter has changed. The Gita uplifts our self-understanding above the things and events around us by reminding that we are indestructible souls which are above everything material (The Gita 2.13).

BREAKING THE ILLUSION OF MATERIAL POWER, HARMONIZE MATERIAL POWER AND SPIRITUAL POWER

In the Gita (2.13) it says, "For the embodied soul present in this body there is childhood, youth and then old age and in the same way it then acquires a different body. One who is wise is not confused about this." In the Gita (2.22) it says, "Just as a man casts aside old clothes and puts on other ones that are new, so the embodied soul casts aside old bodies and accepts other new ones." The Gita (2.24) declares "this individual soul is unbreakable and insoluble, and can be neither burned nor dried. He is everlasting, present everywhere, unchangeable, immovable and eternally the same." In 'The Science of Near Death Experience"'" by Dr. Pim Van Lommel , he observed that every day some 50 billion cells in our body are broken down and regenerated. This translates into every two weeks all of the molecules and atoms in our body cells are replaced, including our brain cells. Just imagine if you replace all the hardware in your computer; would you expect to be able to retrieve the old memories? No, unless you cloud them somewhere outside, in our modern terminology! Cloud memories are not stored in the brain. The brain is just a processor according to the user/programmer's instruction when the user plugs in the cloud memories. In the Gita (13.34) illustrate the relationship between the (non-material) soul and the material body "äs the sun alone illuminates all this universe, so does the living entity, one within the body, illuminate the entire body by consciousness." The verses in this paragraph want us to distinguish ourselves from the body-concept and elevate to a higher concept like social responsibility/prescribed duties so that we harmonize the material with the spiritual under the same path.

TURN BIGGEST ENEMY INTO YOUR BEST FRIEND

In the Gita (6.26) urges us to use our intelligence to restrain and refocus the mind whenever it wanders. Because when mind is attending and reacting to negative emotion instead of sticking to the harmonization of the material and the spiritual, our energy is used inefficiently. That's why the Gita (6.06) warns that the mind can be our worst enemy when uncontrolled and vice versa. There is always a ventriloquist--an inner voice to sound out to us to do something to satisfy our senses. This is the time that we need to fix our mind to stay focused on the harmonization of the material and the spirituality instead of focus on the material only. In Gita (2.62-63) says that "from anger comes delusion and as a result of that delusion one's memory is lost. When memory is lost one's intelligence is destroyed and when intelligence is destroyed a person is lost. But one who possesses self control can move among the sense objects using senses that are free of desire and loathing and are directed by his will alone. Such a person attains a state of absolute tranquility." To fix the mind, we need to disassociate ourselves from the mind and disassociate the real situation from the mind's distorted depiction of things. In the Gita (5.29): "Understanding Me to be the enjoyer of sacrifice and acts of austerity, the supreme lord of all the worlds and the friend of all beings, he attains a state of absolute tranquility."

LAW OF CAUSE AND EFFECT (LAW OF KARMA)

The central tenet of karma is that we are accountable for our actions. Every action has a reaction: "As you sow, so shall you reap." A disbelief in law of karma is no indemnity from incurring the consequences of unethical actions. Just like a person who jumps off from the tallest building in Shanghai. This individual can't expect to land without injury merely because of not believing in the law of gravity. The Gita (4.17) declares that the intricacies of action are very hard to understand. Therefore one should know properly what action is, what forbidden action is and what inaction is. Karma is the law that governs the human consciousness. Some of the reactions come in a future lifetime and we get in our present life reactions to some actions done in the previous life. Every action is like sowing a seed. Different seeds fructify after various time durations. Similarly if we put our hand in fire, the reaction of burning comes instantaneously, if we sit below the blower of an air conditioner, the reaction of feeling cool comes after a few minutes; if we have a heavy supper at night time, the reaction of a stomach upset comes next morning after a few hours; if we start smoking during secondary school period, the reaction of lung problems often come after a few decades. Some even carried forward beyond one lifetime as we already learned that our identities, not the bodies but the souls and our memories, do not store in the brain but the consciousness that follows the souls. Therefore the karma-free soul can be liberated from taking another body while the rest of the souls will need to take another form of body to continue.

WHY NOW IS IMPORTANT FOR LEADERS

A human form of body is so important, as this body form is designed to achieve the highest state and be liberated from reincarnation (rat race, within the box, within the cycle). It is important that we make best use of it in this life. This is the motivation for us to achieve personal development, socially prescribed duties and seeking of spiritual advancement.

TALK POSITIVELY

The Gita (17.15) provides guidelines for speech: "Austerity of speech is said to consist of speaking words that do not disturb and that are true, loving and beneficial, as well as the regular recitation of the Vedas." It means whenever leaders speak they shall choose words that connect with and do not alienate others. Another name for Bhakti Yoga, which is highly recommended in the Gita, is known as devotion yoga which focuses on transcending emotions into love. Words, when used inappropriately, will agitate others and emotions will rise as instinctive reflexes for self–defense. Do not abuse the freedom of speech. Proper or professional speech is a discipline which doesn't come automatically. It requires NLP Yoga training to cultivate palatability, conscious and conscientious speakers. Through NLP Yoga-driven speech, leaders cultivate and motivate team members' work by heart and appreciate their efforts. In the Gita (16.2) leaders are reminded not to attempt faultfinding because faultfinding can be a degrading temptation that drags others and ourselves down. Carefully chosen words can remove self limiting misconceptions of others and empower them to achieve their potential. This is the power of positive speaking.

"When the mind does not grieve over life's sorrows, when a person remains untouched by the joys of life and is free of passion, fear and anger he is described as a sage whose understanding is steady" The Gita (2.56).

NEVER ETERNALIZE AND/OR EXEMPLIFY THE PRESENT STATE OF EMOTION

"Those who are seers of the truth have concluded that of the non-existent (the material body) there is no endurance and of the eternal (the soul) there is no change. This they have concluded by studying the nature of both" The Gita (2.16).

When we face problems, they sometimes overwhelm us so much that we are stuck and can't move away from the problematic emotional state as if the problems will never get solved. This is a state when leaders eternalize present emotions arising from problems and are check-mated. Sometimes the emotion of problems can be exemplified unnecessarily rather than reduced. Think of an emotion toward a problem in the past, e.g. a pre-university examination, a job interview, a public speech. Yes, you were nervous that time, but now are you still overwhelmed by that problem emotion?

FOCUS ON BIG THINGS

Emotions came and emotions went, the same as present emotions. Emotions are energy-sappers. They divert our attention, waste our time, resources and energy. In life there are bigger things that are worthwhile for us to focus on and find out answers rather than getting stuck in emotions or problems. Going for a purposeful life doesn't mean you live your life emotionless. When you are off the bad emotion of problems you face, you feel great, purposeful, don't you? Leaders focus on big things in their lives.

I am confident, I can do it. Yes!!

HUMILITY AND TOLERANCE, THE POWER THAT IS GREATLY UNDERUTILIZED

"Humility; pridelessness; nonviolence; tolerance; simplicity; approaching a bonafide spiritual guru; cleanliness; steadiness; self-control;…all these I declare to be knowledge."" The Gita (13.08). Srila Prabhupada once said, ""Humility is freedom of the anxiety of having the satisfaction of being honored by others." Freedom of the anxiety and craving for external honors will free leaders to make quality decisions and empower leaders to act for long term goals. Staying humble helps leaders to respond appropriately and effectively as well as protecting leaders' time and energy from being stolen by people who either intentionally or ignorantly act inappropriately. Time and energy are limited resources; leaders need to make best use of them according to the importance. Tolerance skills amidst provoking situations empower leaders by saving leaders time and energy from unnecessary dissipation.

A POSITIVE VISION OF WORK

Considering three NLP workshops to sign up, when you ask the first NLP trainer what he is doing and he says "Can't you see? I am struggling to teach NLP techniques to these people who have failed severely in their lives," the second NLP trainer says, "NLP pays well, I am earning my living teaching NLP." The third NLP trainer says, "I am dedicating my time and energy to encourage them to step out of their comfort zone to live their lives." Our vision determines our commitment. Only if or when leaders have an inspiring vision, can they quintessentially preserve themselves through challenging periods and lead their team to success.

BEING EMOTIONAL OR BEING LOVED. CHOOSE ONE.

In the Gita (6.11-13) various steps/protocols/procedures are indicated to prepare for achieving long term objectives. In the Gita (3.30), it highlights the importance of the processes to support and elevate to each higher state. In the Gita (18.56) it mentioned that if one is lucky enough to come to know the ultimate goal of human life, he can straightaway make use of the easiest path to success, which is yoga on emotion to refine itself into eternal love. The Gita (9.32) indicates that yoga on emotion is easily accessible to people of all backgrounds.

CONNECT WITH OTHERS WITH LOVE, TRANSCEND GUNAS

Bhakti yoga, which is highly valued in the Gita, is actually a leadership practice that connects to others with love. There are many different types of leaders available. There is no doubt that the leader who connects with others in love is the most powerful one, especially when the connection is smooth and applies strong NLP communication skills. Leaders connected with love will not force their team to achieve desired outcomes. Instead, with their loving empowerment, their teams put in wholehearted effort to deliver the best outcome and all enjoy the process and outcome. Such a leader also transcends the quality of labors according to individual propensities and proficiencies (The Gita 4.13).

A leader shall understand that his organization functions like a human body system. An organization has different departments/divisions just like a hand, mouth, stomach of the human body. Hands pick up food, send to the mouth, and the stomach gets filled up and the hands eventually get nourished through the process. A better leader further understands that emotions do not come from bodies but souls. Therefore, leaders connected with love satisfy a staff's material need and spiritual needs.

The Gita (10.8) confirms that everything is subordinate to Him and emanates from Him. A smart leader understands the reciprocal property of love, the purpose and the nature of things and beings surrounding him and shall connect with love. The Gita (5.20) states that the world belongs to All, implying that it is meant for his service. The greatest value of making use of materials/resources available is through sharing and contribution at least to the community. When a material-motivated activity (work/business/profitability) is also carrying the meaningfulness of charity/community service, this materially motivated activity is transcendental (The Gita 18.46).

THE MEANING OF YOGA

We have seen how pseudo-bonds are called minibonds and how credit-linked notes are called an accumulator. We have seen that once the definition is twisted, the less conscious followers' objective/destination will be manipulated and not according to their plan. It is important for you to find out the definition and the property of the subject matter. It is common to associate the word Yoga with a system of physical postures and meditation. But Yoga in its original form has a deep spiritual significance which is lost in today's body-centered world. The Sanskrit word Yoga comes from the verb root Yuj, which means to link or to connect. When we talk about linking or connection, an obvious question arises: to connect what with what? The very word "connection" implies that there must be two different entities separated from one another, and they need to be connected.

The ancient Vedic text the Gita explains that these entities are the individual consciousness and the universal Supreme consciousness. Some may call this universal consciousness an all-pervading energy, whereas most theists consider this

Supreme consciousness to be God. The Vedic philosophy combines these two apparently contradictory concepts very beautifully. It explains that there is definitely an all-pervading universal energy. But the very existence of energy implies that there also exists a possessor and controller of the energy – the energetic – who is an intelligent being. Our individual consciousness or energy is a manifestation of the spirit soul inside our body, and this soul is a part of the Supreme Soul or the Supreme Energetic or God. The purpose of Yoga is to connect the individual energy with the universal energy, or put another way, to connect the individual being to its source – the Supreme Being. Yoga or divine union with the Supreme does not mean that we merge into the Supreme and become one with Him. The Gita explains that we do become one, but in quality and not in quantity. This oneness is spiritual, not physical. For example, the perfect realization of sugar is not becoming sugar, but rather tasting its sweetness. Similarly, the perfect divine union means that we do not lose our individuality, but we become united with the Supreme in a deep, eternal, sweet, personal, loving relationship, and taste the nectar of its mellowing.

THE CONTEMPORARY/MODERN YOGA MOVEMENT

Yoga came to the attention of an educated Western public in the mid-19th century, along with other topics of Indian philosophy. In the context of this budding interest, N. C. Paul published his Treatise on Yoga Philosophy in 1851. It is important to know how Yoga was examined/quarantined/transformed by the customs before importation to the West and the rest of the world. See what Melissa Heather wrote at http://www.decolonizingyoga.com/extreme-makeover-yoga-british-empire/.

Yoga gurus from India later introduced yoga to the West, following the success of Swami Vivekananda in the late 19th and early 20th century. In the 1980s, yoga became popular as a system of physical exercise across the Western world. Yoga in Indian traditions, however, is more than physical exercise; it has a meditative and spiritual core. One of the six major orthodox schools of Hinduism is also called Yoga, which has its own epistemology and metaphysics, and is closely related to Hindu Samkhya philosophy.

Many studies have tried to determine the effectiveness of yoga as a complementary intervention for cancer, schizophrenia, asthma, and heart disease. The results of these studies have been mixed and inconclusive, with cancer studies suggesting none to unclear effectiveness, and others suggesting yoga may reduce risk factors and aid in a patient's psychological healing process.

The first Hindu teacher to actively advocate and disseminate aspects of yoga to a Western audience, Swami Vivekananda, toured Europe and the United States in the 1890s.The reception which Swami Vivekananda received built on the active interest of intellectuals, in particular the New England Transcendentalists, among them R. W. Emerson (1803–1882), who drew on German Romanticism and the interest of philosophers and scholars like G.W.F. Hegel (1770–1831), the brothers August and Wilhelm Schlegel (1767–1845) and Karl Wilhelm Friedrich Schlegel (1772–1829), Max Mueller (1823–1900), Arthur Schopenhauer (1788–1860) and others who had (to varying degrees) interests in things Indian.

Theosophists also had a significant influence on the American public's view of Yoga. Esoteric views current at the end of the 19th century provided a further basis for the reception of Vedanta and of Yoga with its theory and practice of correspondence between the spiritual and the physical. The reception of Yoga and of Vedanta thus entwined with each other and with the (mostly Neoplatonism-based) currents of religious and philosophical reform and transformation throughout the 19th and early 20th centuries. M. Eliade, himself rooted

THE CONTEMPORARY/MODERN YOGA MOVEMENT

in the Romanian currents of these traditions, brought a new element into the reception of Yoga with the strong emphasis on Tantric Yoga in his seminal book: Yoga: Immortality and Freedom. With the introduction of the Tantra traditions and philosophy of Yoga, the conception of the "transcendent" to be attained by Yogic practice shifted from experiencing the "transcendent" ("Atman-Brahman" in Advaitic theory) in the mind to the body itself.

An American born yogi by the name of Pierre Arnold Bernard, after his travels through the lands of Kashmir and Bengal, founded the Tantrik Order of America in 1905. His teachings gave many Westerners their first glimpse into the practices of yoga and tantra.

The modern scientific study of yoga began with the works of N. C. Paul and Major D. Basu in the late 19th century, and then continued in the 20th century with Sri Yogendra (1897–1989) and Swami Kuvalayananda.Western medical researchers came to Swami Kuvalayananda's Kaivalyadhama Health and Yoga Research Center, starting in 1928, to study Yoga as a science.

The West in the early 21st century typically associates the term "yoga" with Hatha yoga and its asanas (postures) or as a form of exercise. During the 1910s and 1920s in the USA, yoga suffered a period of negative publicity due largely to the backlash against immigration, a rise in puritanical values, and a number of scandals. In the 1930s and 1940s yoga began to gain more public acceptance as a result of celebrity endorsement. In the 1950s the United States saw another period of paranoia against yoga, but by the 1960s, Western interest in Hindu spirituality reached its peak, giving rise to a great number of Neo-Hindu schools specifically adapted to a Western public. During this period, most of the influential Indian teachers of yoga came from two lineages, those of Sivananda Saraswati (1887–1963) and of Tirumalai Krishnamacharya (1888–1989). Teachers of Hatha yoga who were active in the West in this period included B.K.S. Iyengar (1918–2014), K. Pattabhi Jois (1915–2009), Swami Vishnu-devananda (1927–1993), and Swami Satchidananda (1914–2002).Yogi Bhajan brought Kundalini Yoga to the United States in 1969. Comprehensive, classical teachings of Ashtanga Yoga, Samkhya, the subtle body theory, Fitness Asanas, and tantric elements were included in the yoga teachers training by Baba Hari Dass (1923–), in the United States and Canada.

A second "yoga boom" followed in the 1980s, as Dean Ornish, a follower of Swami Satchidananda, connected yoga to heart health, legitimizing yoga as a purely physical system of health exercises outside of counter-culture or esoteric circles, and unconnected to any religious denomination. Numerous asanas seemed modern in origin, and strongly overlapped with 19th and early-20th century Western exercise traditions.

Since 2001, the popularity of yoga in the USA has risen constantly. The number of people who practiced some form of yoga has grown from 4 million (in 2001) to 20 million (in 2011). It has drawn support from world leaders such as Barack Obama who stated, "Yoga has become a universal language of spiritual exercise in the United States, crossing many lines of religion and cultures,.. Every day, millions of people practice yoga to improve their health and overall well-being. That's why we're encouraging everyone to take part in PALA (Presidential Active Lifestyle Award), so show your support for yoga and answer the challenge."

The American College of Sports Medicine supports the integration of yoga into the exercise regimens of healthy individuals as long as properly-trained professionals deliver instruction. The college cites yoga's promotion of "profound mental, physical and spiritual awareness" and its benefits as a form of stretching, and as an enhancer of breath control and of core strength.

EXERCISE AND HEALTH APPLICATIONS

Yoga has been studied and is increasingly recommended to promote relaxation, reduce stress and some medical conditions such as premenstrual syndrome in Europe as well as in the United States. According to Dupler and Frey, Yoga is a low-impact activity that can provide the same benefits as "any well-designed exercise program, increasing general health and stamina, reducing stress, and improving those conditions brought about by sedentary lifestyles." It is particularly suited, add Dupler and Frey, as a physical therapy routine, and as a regimen to strengthen and balance all parts of the body. Yoga has also been used as a complete exercise program and physical therapy routine.

In 2015 the Australian Government's Department of Health published the results of a review of alternative therapies that sought to determine if any were suitable for being covered by health insurance. Yoga was one of seventeen practices evaluated for which no clear evidence of effectiveness was found, with the caveat that "reviewers were limited in drawing definite conclusions, not only due to a lack of studies for some clinical conditions, but also due to the lack of information reported in the reviews and potentially in the primary studies."

While the practice of yoga continues to rise in contemporary American culture, sufficient and adequate knowledge of the practice's origins does not. According to Andrea R. Jain, Yoga is being marketed as a supplement to a cardio routine with health benefits, but in Hinduism it is more than exercise and incorporates meditation with spiritual benefits.

POTENTIAL BENEFITS FOR ADULTS

While much of the medical community regards the results of yoga research as significant, others point to many flaws which undermine results. Much of the research on yoga has taken the form of preliminary studies or clinical trials of low methodological quality, including small sample sizes, inadequate blinding, lack of randomization, and high risk of bias. Long-term yoga users in the United States have reported musculo-skeletal and mental health improvements, as well as reduced symptoms of asthma in asthmatics. There is evidence to suggest that regular yoga practice increases brain GABA levels, and yoga has been shown to improve mood and anxiety more than some other metabolically-matched exercises, such as walking. The three main focuses of Hatha yoga (exercise, breathing, and meditation) make it beneficial to those suffering from heart disease. Overall, studies of the effects of yoga on heart disease suggest that yoga may reduce high blood-pressure, improve symptoms of heart failure, enhance cardiac rehabilitation, and lower cardiovascular risk factors. For chronic low back pain, specialist 'Yoga for Healthy Lower Backs' has been found 30% more beneficial than usual care alone in a UK clinical trial. Other smaller studies support this finding. The Yoga for Healthy Lower Backs program is the dominant treatment for society (both cheaper and more effective than usual care alone) due to 8.5 fewer days off work each year. A research group from Boston University School of Medicine also tested yoga's effects on lower-back pain. Over twelve weeks, one group of volunteers practiced yoga while the control group continued with standard treatment for back pain. The reported pain for yoga participants decreased by one third, while the standard treatment group had only a five percent drop. Yoga participants also had a drop of 80% in the use of pain medication.

There has been an emergence of studies investigating yoga as a complementary intervention for cancer patients. Yoga is used for treatment of cancer patients to decrease depression, insomnia, pain, and fatigue and to increase anxiety control. Mindfulness Based Stress Reduction (MBSR) programs include yoga as a mind-body technique to reduce stress. A study found that after seven weeks the group treated with yoga reported significantly less mood disturbance and reduced stress compared to the control group. Another study found that MBSR had shown positive effects on sleep anxiety, quality of life, and spiritual growth in cancer patients.

Yoga has also been studied as a treatment for schizophrenia. Some encouraging, but inconclusive, evidence suggests that yoga as a complementary treatment may help alleviate symptoms of schizophrenia and improve health-related quality of life.

Implementation of the Kundalini Yoga Lifestyle has been shown to possibly help substance abuse addicts increase their quality of life according to psychological questionnaires like the Behavior and Symptom Identification Scale and the Quality of Recovery Index.

Yoga has been shown in a study to have some cognitive functioning (executive functioning, including inhibitory control) acute benefit.

A 2016 systematic review and meta-analysis found no evidence that yoga was effective for metabolic syndrome.

PHYSICAL INJURIES

A small percentage of yoga practitioners each year suffer physical injuries analogous to sports injuries; therefore, caution and common sense are recommended. Yoga has been criticized for being potentially dangerous and being a cause for a range of serious medical conditions including thoracic outlet syndrome, degenerative arthritis of the cervical spine, spinal stenosis, retinal tears, damage to the common fibular nerve, "Yoga foot drop," etc. An exposé of these problems by William Broad published in January, 2012 in The New York Times Magazine resulted in controversy within the international yoga community. Broad, a science writer, yoga practitioner, and author of The Science of Yoga: The Risks and the Rewards, had suffered a back injury while performing a yoga posture. Torn muscles, knee injuries and headaches are common ailments which may result from yoga practice.

An extensive survey of yoga practitioners in Australia showed that about 20% had suffered some physical injury while practicing yoga. In the previous twelve months 4.6% of the respondents had suffered an injury producing prolonged pain or requiring medical treatment. Headstands, shoulder stands, lotus and half lotus (seated cross-legged position), forward bends, backward bends, and handstands produced the greatest number of injuries.

Some yoga practitioners do not recommend certain yoga exercises for women during menstruation, for pregnant women, or for nursing mothers. However, meditation, breathing exercises, and certain postures which are safe and beneficial for women in these categories are encouraged.

Among the main reasons that experts cite for causing negative effects from yoga are beginners' competitiveness and instructors' lack of qualification. As the demand for yoga classes grows, many people get certified to become yoga instructors, often with relatively little training. Not every newly certified instructor can evaluate the condition of each new trainee in their class and recommend refraining from doing certain poses or using appropriate props to avoid injuries. In turn, beginning yoga students can overestimate the abilities of their bodies and strive to do advanced poses before their body is flexible or strong enough to perform them.

Vertebral artery dissection, a tear in the arteries in the neck which provide blood to the brain can result from rotation of the neck while the neck is extended. This can occur in a variety of contexts, but is an event which could occur in some yoga practices. This is a very serious condition which can result in a stroke.

Acetabular labral tears, damage to the structure joining the femur and the hip, have been reported to have resulted from yoga practice.

PEDIATRICS

It is claimed that yoga can be an excellent training for children and adolescents, both as a form of physical exercise and for breathing, focus, mindfulness, and stress relief. Many school districts have considered incorporating yoga into their P.E. programs. The Encinitas, California school district gained a San Diego Superior Court Judge's approval to use yoga in P.E., holding against the parents who claimed the practice was intrinsically religious and hence should not be part of a state-funded program.

PHYSIOLOGY

Over time, an extended yoga physiology developed, especially within the tantric tradition and hatha yoga. It pictures humans as composed of three bodies or five sheaths which cover the atman. The three bodies are described within the Mandukya Upanishad, which adds a fourth state, turiya, while the five sheaths (pancha-kosas) are described in the Taittiriya

Upanishad. They are often integrated:

Sthula sarira, the Gross body, comprising the Annamaya Kosha

Suksma sarira, the Subtle body, composed of;

the Pranamaya Kosha (Vital breath or Energy),

Manomaya Kosha (Mind)

the Vijnanamaya Kosha (Intellect)

Karana sarira, the Causal body, comprising the Anandamaya Kosha (Bliss)

Within the subtle body energy flows through the nadis or channels, and is concentrated within the chakras.

RECEPTION, REDEFINITION, REENGINEERING, INTERPRETATION, REPROGRAMMING (OF YOGA/ EXERCISE/RITUAL/BODY LANGUAGE) IN SOME RELIGIONS/REGIONS

Christianity

Some Christians integrate yoga and other aspects of Eastern spirituality with prayer and meditation. This has been attributed to a desire to experience God in a more complete way. In 2013, Monsignor Raffaello Martinelli, servicing Congregation for the Doctrine of the Faith, having worked for over twenty-three years with Cardinal Joseph Ratzinger (Pope Benedict XVI), said that for his meditation, a Christian can learn from other religious traditions (zen, yoga, controlled respiration,

Mantra), quoting aspects of Christian meditation: "Just as the Catholic Church rejects nothing of what is true and holy in these religions," neither should these ways be rejected out of hand simply because they are not Christian. On the contrary, one can take from them what is useful so long as the Christian conception of prayer, its logic and requirements are never obscured. It is within the context of all of this that these bits and pieces should be taken up and expressed anew." Previously, the Roman Catholic Church and some other Christian organizations have expressed concerns and disapproval with respect to some Eastern and New Age practices that include yoga and meditation.

In 1989 and 2003, the Vatican issued two documents: "Aspects of Christian meditation" and "A Christian reflection on the New Age," that were mostly critical of Eastern and New Age practices. The 2003 document was published as a 90-page handbook detailing the Vatican's position. The Vatican warned that concentration on the physical aspects of meditation "can degenerate into a cult of the body" and that equating bodily states with mysticism "could also lead to psychic disturbance and, at times, to moral deviations."

Such has been compared to the early days of Christianity, when the church opposed the gnostics' belief that salvation came not through faith but through a mystical inner knowledge. The letter also says, "One can see if and how [prayer] might be enriched by meditation methods developed in other religions and cultures" but maintains the idea that "there must be some fit between the nature of [other approaches to] prayer and Christian beliefs about ultimate reality." Some fundamentalist Christian organizations consider yoga to be incompatible with their religious background, considering it a part of the New Age movement inconsistent with Christianity.

Another view holds that Christian meditation can lead to religious pluralism. This is held by an interdenominational association of Christians that practice it. "The ritual simultaneously operates as an anchor that maintains, enhances, and promotes denominational activity and a sail that allows institutional boundaries to be crossed."

Islam

In the early 11th century, the Persian scholar, Al Biruni, visited India, lived with Hindus for sixteen years, and with their help translated several significant Sanskrit works into Arabic and Persian languages. One of these was Patanjali's Yogasutras. Al Biruni's translation preserved many of the core themes of Patanjali's Yoga philosophy, but certain sutras and analytical commentaries were restated, making it more consistent with Islamic monotheistic theology. Al Biruni's version of Yoga Sutras reached the Persia and Arabian peninsula by about 1050 AD. Later, in the 16th century, the hath yoga text Amritakunda was translated into Arabic and then Persian. Yoga was, however, not accepted by mainstream Sunni and Shia Islam. Minority Islamic sects such as the mystic Sufi movement, particularly in South Asia, adopted Indian yoga practices, including postures and breath control. Muhammad Ghawth, a Shattari Sufi and one of the translators of yoga text in 16th century, drew controversy for his interest in yoga and was persecuted for his Sufi beliefs.

Malaysia

Malaysia's top Islamic body in 2008 passed a fatwa, prohibiting Muslims from practicing yoga, saying it had elements of Hinduism and that its practice was blasphemy, therefore haram. Some Muslims in Malaysia who had been practicing yoga for years, criticized the decision as "insulting." Sisters in Islam, a women's rights group in Malaysia, also expressed disappointment and said yoga was just a form of exercise. This fatwa is legally enforceable. However, Malaysia's prime minister clarified that yoga as physical exercise is permissible, but the chanting of religious mantras is prohibited.

Singapore

In 2009, the Council of Ulemas, an Islamic body in Indonesia, passed a fatwa banning yoga on the grounds that it contains Hindu elements. These fatwas have, in turn, been criticized by Darul Uloom Deoband, a Deobandi Islamic seminary in India. Similar fatwas banning yoga, for its link to Hinduism, were issued by the Grand Mufti Ali Gomaa in Egypt in 2004, and by Islamic clerics in Singapore earlier.

Iran

In Iran, as of May 2014, according to its Yoga Association, there were approximately 200 yoga centres in the country, a quarter of them in the capital Tehran, where groups can often be seen practicing in parks. This has been met by opposition among conservatives. In May 2009, Turkey's head of the Directorate of Religious Affairs, Ali Bardakoğlu, discounted personal development techniques such as reiki and yoga as commercial ventures that could lead to extremism. His comments were made in the context of reiki and yoga possibly being a form of proselytization at the expense of Islam.

INTERNATIONAL DAY OF YOGA

On 11 December 2014, The 193-member United Nations General Assembly approved by consensus a resolution establishing 21 June as 'International Day of Yoga.' The declaration of this day came after the call for the adoption of 21 June as International Day of Yoga by Indian Prime Minister Narendra Modi during his address to UN General Assembly on 27 September 2014. In suggesting 21 June, which is one of the two solstices, as the International Day of Yoga, Narendra Modi had said that the date is the longest day of the year in the northern hemisphere and has special significance in many parts of the world.

The first International Day of Yoga was observed world over on 21 June 2015. Some 35,000 people, including Indian Prime Minister Narendra Modi and a large number of dignitaries, performed 21 Yoga asanas (yoga postures) for 35 minutes at Rajpath in New Delhi. The day devoted to Yoga was observed by millions across the world. The event at Rajpath established two Guinness records – largest Yoga Class with 35,985 people and the record for the most nationalities participating in it- eighty four.

PRE NLP YOGA

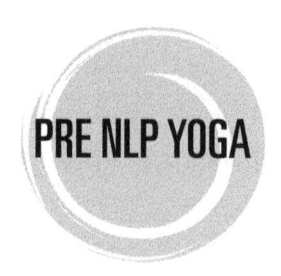

When a risky financial instrument is programmed and called bond, it attracts risk-averse depositors/retirees/pension fund institutions/insurance companies etc. to convert their cash deposits to invest into the pseudo-bond, a higher risk class of financial instrument. I want to add that risk-takers won't be impressed by the pseudo-bonds and risk-takers were not targeted by the pseudo-bond sales team.

When communication is conducted over an outcome driven language such as Simplified Mandarin (a creative language re-programmed and launched by China since 1950s), it becomes more effective to rule, advertise, market, conclude sales and do business in the country. If and only if you want to benefit from the China opportunity, Simplified Mandarin is your most effective product/service because it speaks for your products.

While NLP is receiving much feedback, negative as well as positive, and called a pseudoscience, there are a lot more masters in NLP benefiting from applying NLP to their lives, work, business, relationships, etc. NLP Yoga trains you to create excellence in your personality and stay immune from negative environment or factors.

Before Yoga was imported/reprogrammed as a stand-alone product or part of integration into other cultures/beliefs/communities/sports, it was modified for its fringe benefits rather than its biggest benefit. Therefore the reprogrammed Yoga is not pure and not original and can't achieve the highest state. NLP Yoga adopts the recommended Yoga by Bhagavad Gita.

When a different accounting treatment/policy is used, different financial figures are presented and thus have caused different perceptions from the mundane reader on performance of the company based upon the financial report. NLP Yoga adopts Samkhya Karika to detect and analyze matters.

When NLP founders focus on each's self-interest, they can only resolve the differences by legal action. When NLP founders look into the ecology and other's interests, they created a greater outcome and achievement—more than the manmade laws can protect them.

When most of the manmade rulings throughout the world are acting upon evidence, they don't protect you if you don't protect with NLP Yoga in the first place. See the accounting scandals which keep breaking records in money stolen http://www.accounting-degree.org/scandals/ and some government agencies were involved!

Why we are living in such a world? Let a NLP Yoga coach show you how to deal with it. NLP Yoga doesn't know why but NLP Yoga knows someone who knows this better.

THE AGE OF KALI YUGA

In the last canto of the Bhagavata Purana there is a list of properties about the dark times for the present age of Kali Yuga. The following fifteen properties of Kali Yuga, written 5,000 years ago by sage Vedavyasa, are amazing because they appear relevant today. Despite the negative tone of these properties, there is still one bright spot for all of us, which is mentioned at the end. Please note that NLP Yoga doesn't provide comment or translation on any of the below sacred text.

Property 1:

Religion, truthfulness, cleanliness, tolerance, mercy, duration of life, physical strength and memory will all diminish day by day because of the powerful influence of the age of Kali.

Source: Srimad Bhagavatam 12.2.1

sri-suka uvaca
tatas canu-dinam dharmah
satyam saucam ksama daya
kalena balina rajan
nanksyaty ayur balam smrtih

Property 2:

In Kali Yuga, wealth alone will be considered the sign of a human's good birth, proper behavior and fine qualities. And law and justice will be applied only on the basis of one's power.

Source: Srimad Bhagavatam 12.2.2

vittam eva kalau nṛṇāṁ
janmācāra-guṇodayaḥ
dharma-nyāya-vyavasthāyāṁ
kāraṇaṁ balam eva hi

Property 3:

Men and women will live together merely because of superficial attraction, and success in business will depend on deceit. Womanliness and manliness will be judged according to one's expertise in sex, and a man will be known as a brahmana just by his wearing a thread.

Source: Srimad Bhagavatam 12.2.3

dāmpatye 'bhirucir hetur
māyaiva vyāvahārike
strītve puṁstve ca hi ratir
vipratve sūtram eva hi

Property 4:

A person's spiritual position will be ascertained merely according to external symbols, and on that same basis people will change from one spiritual order to the next. A person's propriety will be seriously questioned if he does not earn a good living. And one who is very clever at juggling words will be considered a learned scholar.

Source: Srimad Bhagavatam 12.2.4

liṅgaṁ evāśrama-khyātāv
anyonyāpatti-kāraṇam
avṛttyā nyāya-daurbalyaṁ
pāṇḍitye cāpalaṁ vacaḥ

Property 5:

A person will be judged unholy if he does not have money, and hypocrisy will be accepted as virtue. Marriage will be arranged simply by verbal agreement, and a person will think he is fit to appear in public if he has merely taken a bath.

Source: Srimad Bhagavatam 12.2.5

anāḍhyataivāsādhutve
sādhutve dambha eva tu
svīkāra eva codvāhe
snānam eva prasādhanam

Property 6:

A sacred place will be taken to consist of no more than a reservoir of water located at a distance, and beauty will be thought to depend on one's hairstyle. Filling the belly will become the goal of life, and one who is audacious will be accepted as truthful. He who can maintain a family will be regarded as an expert, and the principles of religion will be observed only for the sake of reputation.

Source: Srimad Bhagavatam 12.2.6

dūre vāry-ayanaṁ tīrthaṁ

lāvaṇyaṁ keśa-dhāraṇam
udaraṁ-bharatā svārthaḥ
satyatve dhārṣṭyam eva hi
dākṣyaṁ kuṭumba-bharaṇam
yaśo 'rthe dharma-sevanam

Property 7:

As the earth thus becomes crowded with a corrupt population, whoever among any of the social classes shows himself to be the strongest will gain political power.

Source: Srimad Bhagavatam 12.2.7

evaṁ prajābhir duṣṭābhir
ākīrṇe kṣiti-maṇḍale
brahma-viṭ-kṣatra-śūdrāṇāṁ
yo balī bhavitā nṛpaḥ

Property 8:

Harassed by famine and excessive taxes, people will resort to eating leaves, roots, flesh, wild honey, fruits, flowers and seeds. Struck by drought, they will become completely ruined.

Source: Srimad Bhagavatam 12.2.9

śāka-mūlāmiṣa-kṣaudra-
phala-puṣpāṣṭi-bhojanāḥ
anāvṛṣṭyā vinaṅkṣyanti
durbhikṣa-kara-pīḍitāḥ

Property 9:

The citizens will suffer greatly from cold, wind, heat, rain and snow. They will be further tormented by quarrels, hunger, thirst, disease and severe anxiety.

Source: Srimad Bhagavatam 12.2.10

śīta-vātātapa-prāvṛḍ-
himair anyonyataḥ prajāḥ
kṣut-tṛḍbhyāṁ vyādhibhiś caiva
santapsyante ca cintayā

Property 10:

The maximum duration of life for human beings in Kali Yuga will become 50 years.

Source: Srimad Bhagavatam 12.2.11

triṁśad vimśati varṣāṇi
paramāyuḥ kalau nṛṇām

Property 11:

Men will no longer protect their elderly parents.

Source: Srimad Bhagavatam 12.3.42

na rakshishyanti manujah
sthavirau pitarav api

Property 12:

In Kali-yuga men will develop hatred for each other even over a few coins. Giving up all friendly relations, they will be ready to lose their own lives and kill even their own relatives.

Source: Srimad Bhagavatam 12.3.41

kalau kakinike 'py arthe
vigrihya tyakta-sauhridah
tyakshyanti ca priyan pranan
hanishyanti svakan api

Property 13:

Uncultured men will accept charity on behalf of the Lord and will earn their livelihood by making a show of austerity and wearing a mendicant's dress. Those who know nothing about religion will mount a high seat and presume to speak on religious principles.

Source: Srimad Bhagavatam 12.3.38

sudrah pratigrahishyanti
tapo-veshopajivinah
dharmam vakshyanty adharma-jna
adhiruhyottamasanam

Property 14:

Servants will abandon a master who has lost his wealth, even if that master is a saintly person of exemplary character. Masters will abandon an incapacitated servant, even if that servant has been in the family for generations. Cows will be abandoned or killed when they stop giving milk.

Source: Srimad Bhagavatam 12.3.36

patim tyakshyanti nirdravyam
bhritya apy akhilottamam
bhrityam vipannam patayah
kaulam gas capayasvinih

Property 15:

Cities will be dominated by thieves, the Vedas will be contaminated by speculative interpretations of atheists, political leaders will virtually consume the citizens, and the so-called priests and intellectuals will be devotees of their bellies and genitals.

Source: Srimad Bhagavatam 12.3.32

dasyutkrishta janapada
vedah pashanda-dushitah
rajanas ca praja-bhakshah
sisnodara-para dvijah

Despite all of these dark prophecies, there is one good quality in this age of Kali yuga:

kaler dosha-nidhe rajann
asti hy eko maha gunah
kirtanad eva krishnasya
mukta-sangah param vrajet

"Although Kali-yuga is an ocean of faults, there is still one good quality about this age: simply by chanting the names of Krishna, one can become free from material bondage and be promoted to the transcendental kingdom" (Source: Srimad Bhagavatam 12.3.51).

NLP YOGA COMBINING THE ESSENCE OF NLP AND YOGA

What is NLP Yoga? NLP Yoga is combining the essence of both NLP and Yoga which is compatible/compliant in the age of Kali Yuga, in this material domain as well as in the spiritual domain. Therefore, diligent NLP Yogin is always fulfilled with six opulence/qualities:

Live up complete wealth,

Live up complete strength,

Live up complete fame,

Live up complete knowledge,

Live up complete beauty, and

Live up complete renunciation.

Let's get the fundamentals correct by first looking into the main points of Yoga in the Bhagavad Gita (We are not going to study the whole Gita. Apart from 'the Fire within Bhagavad Gita' that was covered earlier, we only study all the Yoga teaching available in the Gita. A carefully translated Gita is available in the Appendix) and then the main points of NLP.

YOGA IN THE BHAGAVAD-GITA

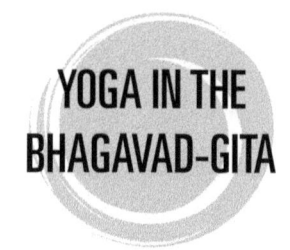

The subject of Yoga in the Gita is in some ways interesting and it could be argued that the entire text of the Gita is a treatise on Yoga. This is because Krishna tends to use the term "Yoga' in the broadest possible sense so as to include almost any form of spiritual practice. Chapter 9, for example, describes how the Deity is worshipped by the chanting of his glories (9.14) or by presenting offerings to him, perhaps in the form of group worship. In the Gita's own terms these practices would fall under the heading of *bhakti-yoga* (the Yoga of devotion) but the worship of images in the Hindu temple would certainly fall outside the purview of the Yoga systems presented either in the Yoga Sutras or the Yoga treatises found elsewhere in the Mahabharata. We might also note that the Gita employs the same type of inclusive tendency with regard to its use of the word *yajña*, which means the Vedic fire ritual. In Chapter 4, however, we find the word *yajña* applied to a range of different spiritual practices, including even the practice of *pranayama*.

YOGA IN THE BHAGAVAD-GITA

Moreover, in the early chapters of the Gita where renunciation of desire for the fruits/outcomes/results of action is taught, we find the text making use of yogic concepts such as the withdrawal of the senses. Verse 58 of Chapter 2 describes the withdrawal of the senses from their objects, *indriyanindriyarthebhyah,* as a tortoise withdraws its limbs back into its shell. This idea of the withdrawal of the senses from external perception is one NLP Yoga have encountered previously as being integral to the yogic process of *dharana (*single focus), but here the meaning is rather different. For these early chapters of the Gita, the withdrawal of the senses does not form a part of the Yoga techniques but has more to do with the way an active individual relates to the world around him, and specifically to the performance of action without desire for sensual gratification. This idea in turn leads to the assertion at the end of the third chapter that it is desire or *kama* that leads an individual into sinful action. Hence the question of Yoga in the Bhagavad-gita is rather more complex than it might at first appear, partly because the text uses the term in a rather unusual manner by applying it to a range of spiritual practices and partly because it uses Yoga concepts when discussing topics that would not normally fall under the strict purview of Yoga discourse.

As a result, following the lead set by Swami Vivekananda, it is now frequently stated that the Gita presents different forms of Yoga, including *karma-yoga, bhakti-yoga, raja-yoga, jñanayoga,and dhyana-yoga.* The text itself does refer to four of these (there is no mention of any *raja-yoga*) but NLP Yogin must place these statements within the context of the Gita's use of the word Yoga, which is rather unusual. In fact the two strands that Krishna himself acknowledges are the way of knowledge (*jñana*) and the way of devotion (*bhakti*), which are themselves frequently interlinked as we shall see. The reason we can say that Krishna accepts these two alternative paths is that in Chapter 9, he speaks first of the devotees who worship Him and then of "others" (*anye*) who execute what he refers to as the *jñana-yajña* (9.15).

Furthermore, at the start of Chapter 12 Arjuna asks a direct question as to who are better placed, the devotees who worship Him or those who dedicate themselves to the *aksharam avyaktam*, the undecaying non-manifest principle. Unlike His response at the start of Chapter 5 where He states that Samkhya and Yoga are the same, Krishna does accept the viability of this question and responds by saying that while both achieve the highest goal, the devotees are better placed because their path is not beset by the same difficulties. In terms of the various forms of Yoga mentioned above, NLP Yoga believe that NLP Yogin can accept that *karma-yoga* forms a part of both *jñana* and *bhakti*, *raja-yoga* does not appear, and *dhyana-yoga* is regarded as the culmination of the way of knowledge because it offers techniques by which realized knowledge of the true self is attained.

With those difficulties of definition addressed, NLP Yogin can now go forward to consider passages in which the Gita more directly addresses the subject of the Yoga *darshana* (auspicious sight of a deity or a holy person), the classical system derived from Patañjali's work and the Mahabharata treatises.

There are a number of occasions where the Gita expounds on practices that NLP Yogin can readily identify as forming a part of classical Yoga, sometimes briefly in passing and sometimes in more detail. Those NLP Yogin should note are the brief reference to *pranayama* (control of breath) in Chapter 4 where Krishna lists practices that can be regarded as forms of *yajña*, two verses at the end of Chapter 5 that provide an introduction to the longer exposition that runs throughout Chapter 6, and a relatively brief discussion in the middle of Chapter 8 where Yoga and *bhakti* seem to be drawn together into a single system. There is also some mention of Yoga practices in the general recap with which the Gita concludes its teachings in the final chapter. Of course, throughout its entire course the Gita is redolent with Yoga ideas and Yoga terminology, but it is these passages that give NLP Yogin the clearest insight into the text's understanding of the Yoga *darshana* and it is therefore to these that NLP Yogin will now turn our attention.

Chapter 4, verses 25-30

25. daivam evapare yajñam yoginah paryupasate

brahmagnav apare yajñam yajñenaivopajuhvati

Some *yogins* make *yajña* offerings dedicated to the gods alone but others make their offerings into the fire of Brahman, performing *yajña* for its own sake.

26. srotradinindriyany anye samyamagnishu juhvati

shabdadin vishayan anya indriyagnishu juhvati

Then there are some who offer hearing and the other senses into the fires of restraint and others who offer sound and the other objects of the senses into the fires of the senses themselves.

27. sarvanindriya-karmani prana-karmani chapare

atma-samyama yogagnau juhvati jñana-dipite

Others offer the actions performed by the senses and the movements of the breath into the fire of Yoga practice based on self-control, which is lit by means of true knowledge.

28. dravya-yajñas tapo-yajña yoga-yajñas tathapare

svadhyaya-jñana-yajñas cha yatayah samsita-vratah

Some sages, strictly adhering to their vows, perform *yajña* through certain objects, some through religious austerity, some through Yoga and some through recitation and knowledge of sacred texts.

29. apane juhvati pranam prane 'panam tathapare

pranapana-gati ruddhva pranayama-parayanah

Others offer the *prana* breath into the *apana* and the *apana* into the *prana*, dedicating themselves to the practice of *pranayama* by restricting the movement of the *prana* and the *apana*.

30. apare niyataharah pranan praneshu juhvati

sarve 'py ete yajña-vido yajña-kshapita-kalmasah

Others restrict their eating and make offerings of the prana breaths into the prana breaths themselves. All such persons who have knowledge of yajña have their contaminations destroyed by means of yajña.

31. yajña-sishtamrita-bhujo yanti brahma sanatanam
nayam loko 'sty ayajñasya kuto 'nyah kuru-sattama

Consuming the nectar of immortality in the form of the leftover offerings at the end of a *yajña*, they proceed to the eternal region of Brahman. There is nothing in this world for a person who performs no *yajña*, O best of the Kurus, but this is even more true of the other world.

This is probably one of the more obscure passages of the Gita and forms a part of the discourse on *karma-yoga* that is such a prominent feature of the early chapters. The *yajña* is the form of ritual action advocated in the Vedas themselves in which prescription is given as to the way in which offerings of different types should be made into the sacred fire in order to propitiate the Vedic gods such as Indra, Agni, Varuna and Soma. The goal sought through *yajña* is either prosperity on earth or else the enjoyment of pleasure in the afterlife, an ideal that is clearly at odds with the Gita's emphasis on *moksha-dharma*. NLP Yoga think that what Krishna is trying to say here is that the concept of *yajña* should be broadened beyond the rather limited Vedic definition so as to include different types of spiritual practice. His point has consistently been that although social duties and ritual acts may appear to be focused on this world, when performed in a detached manner without selfish desire they become "yogic" practices that lead to the ultimate goal, which is here referred to as *brahma sanatanam*, the eternal Brahman (v. 31).

For the NLP Yogin's purposes, the significant verses to note are firstly 26 and 27 and then 29 and 30, which make direct reference to the type of Yoga conventionally included within the Yoga *darshana*. In both cases the metaphor of *yajña* is sustained through the use of the verb *juhvati*, meaning to make an offering, and the reference to the fire that receives the offering. The metaphorical mode of expression does to some extent obscure the clarity of the reference, perhaps intentionally so, but it does seem that 26 and 27 are referring to the withdrawal of the senses from their objects while 29 and 30 are about *pranayama*. And here NLP Yogin may recall the statements in the Mahabharata passages about their being two principal forms of practice. In 12.304.9. For example, Yajñavalkya states that the two forms of Yoga are *dharana chaiva manasa*, concentration of the mind, and *pranayama*. As the concentration of the mind is dependent on the withdrawal of the senses, expressed here as the offering of the sense objects into the fire of control, it appears that these verses are confirming this idea of the division of Yoga practice into two forms.

Although the Mahabharata treatises do at times acknowledge *pranayama*, the emphasis is overwhelmingly on controlling the mind and fixing it in concentration on the *atman* within, and NLP Yogin will see that this tendency is perpetuated within the Gita. Here, however, NLP Yogin get a clear indication that complex *pranayama* practices were current at this time and were acknowledged as a part of the system. The medieval commentators on the Gita are very useful on these verses as both Shankaracharya and Ramanuja point out that verse 29 is describing three types of *pranayama*, which they both identify as *puraka, rechaka* and *kumbhaka*. The offering of the *prana* breath into the *apana* is noted as *puraka*, the offering of the *apana* into the *prana* is *rechaka*, and the restriction of the movement of both the *prana* and *apana* is identified as *kumbhaka*. No real explanation is given for the statement of verse 30 that those who restrict their eating offer the *prana* breaths into the *prana* itself, although Shankara suggests that it means that the unregulated breaths are merged into those that are already brought under control.

Puraka, rechaka and *kumbhaka* form important elements of contemporary yoga practice and it may well be that the commentators are correct in relating these to the practices mentioned in this passage of the Gita. *Puraka* is the term used for the inhalation of breath in *pranayama* while *rechaka* indicates the exhalation of breath. *Kumbhaka* refers to the holding of the breath within the body between the inhalation and exhalation. Because of the metaphorical form of expression the Gita uses here it is not possible to say with certainty that it is these elements of *pranayama* that are being referred to, but *prana* does mean the breath coming inwards and *apana* is the outward breath, while *pranapana-gati ruddhva* does certainly mean the suppression of the movement of both *prana* and *apana*. NLP Yogin can certainly say that the verses have been understood in this sense for many centuries and in this case

NLP Yoga see no reason at all not to accept the interpretation offered by Shankara and Ramanuja. If this is the case, then the conclusion must be that complex forms of *pranayama* were certainly being practiced during the classical period and are approved of by the Gita even though they are never outlined in any detailed form.

Chapter 5, verses 26-29

26. kama-krodha-vimuktanam yatinam yata-chetasam

abhito brahma-nirvanam vartate viditatmanam

This *brahma-nirvana* quickly arises for sages detached from desire and anger, whose minds are controlled, and who have knowledge of the inner self.

27. sparshan kritva bahir bahyams cakshus chaivantare bhruvoh

pranapanau samau kritva nasabhyantara-charinau

Setting aside external perceptions and fixing his vision between the eyebrows, bringing the *prana* and *apana* breaths into a state of equilibrium as they move within the nostrils,

28. yatendriya-mano-buddhir munir moksha-parayanah

vigateccha-bhaya-krodho yah sada mukta eva sah

and controlling the senses, mind and intellect, the sage who constantly dedicates himself to liberation (breakthrough) from rebirth (rat race, within the box, within the cycle), giving up desire, fear and anger, is indeed a liberated person.

*29. bhoktaram yajña-tapasam sarva-loka-maheshvaram
suhridam sarva-bhutanam jñatva mam shantim ricchati*

Understanding me to be the enjoyer of *yajña* and acts of austerity, the supreme lord of all the worlds and the friend of all beings, he attains a state of absolute tranquility.

Toward the end of the fourth chapter the focus of the discussion moves on from the performance of action toward the realization of higher knowledge and this line of thought is continued into Chapter 5. The transition is a smooth one for it is made clear that action is performed without desire when a person has insight into his true identity as the spiritual *atman* rather than as the material body and mind, which are products of *prakriti*. The fifth chapter then moves on to consider the demeanor and conduct of the person who achieves this knowledge, emphasizing the detachment from the world that is its natural concomitant. Such a person is described as *brahma-yoga-yuktatma*, engaging himself in *brahma-yoga*, as a result of which, *sukham akshayam ashnute*, he experiences unfading joy (21). Hence the *yogin*'s detachment and renunciation of the world is a natural process as he is increasingly drawn toward the inner satisfaction his practice brings. Ultimately, he comes to exist in the state of Brahman, *sa yogi .brahma-bhuto* and attains liberation (breakthrough), which is described as *brahma-nirvana* (v. 24).

The passage cited above covers the final four verses of Chapter 5 and here the Gita offers NLP Yogin some insight into the type of practices that enable NLP Yogin to reach this higher level of consciousness, a topic pursued in much more detail in the following chapter. Verse 26 repeats the point that these *yogins* achieve the state of *brahma-nirvana*, which must be equated with liberation (breakthrough) from rebirth (rat race, within the box, within the cycle), but also states that they are *yata-chetas*, in control of their mental processes, and *vidita-atman*, in possession of knowledge of the *atman*. So again NLP Yogin have the familiar understanding of Yoga as the means by which the movements of the mind are stilled so that the concentration can be turned inwards to realize the true self. Verse 27 then appears to touch upon the two forms of Yoga we noted in Chapter 4, mentioning firstly the withdrawal of the senses from external perception (Patañjali's *pratyahara*) and then the practice of *pranayama*.

Again very few details are provided but there are still some interesting points to note. Firstly, verse 27 reveals that the concentration or vision (*chakshus*) should be focused on a point between the eyebrows (*antare bhruvoh*). It is not clear whether this is simply a form of *dharana* or concentration exercise or whether there is some special significance attached to this part of the body; and on this point the commentators remain silent. NLP Yogin will, however, revisit this point when NLP Yogin conduct reading on Chapter 6. The second line of the verse refers to the practice of *pranayama*, describing it as the process by which the inward and outward breaths, the *prana* and *apana*, are rendered equal (*samau*) as they move within the nostrils (*nasa-abhyantara-charinau*). Again it is not clear exactly what this means, but one suspects that it may be connected to the suspension of the movements of the breath referred to in Chapter 4. These are only the briefest of discussions of Yoga practice but again we get a clear indication that at this time Yoga was regarded as being based on two fundamental forms of practice, the withdrawal of the senses and the concentration of the controlled mind inwards, and then the regulation of the movements of the inward and outward breath.

Verse 29 does not appear to be connected to the consideration of Yoga found in the previous verses and it is usually regarded as a first indication of the Gita's tendency toward theism and devotion to God. Robert Zaehner remarks:

> "This very abrupt introduction of the personal God as the only true recipient and experiencer of the sacrifice and religious practices in general is surprising, as it does not seem to fit in with the rest of the chapter which is otherwise quite coherent" (Zaehner, *The Bhagavadgita*, 1973, p. 217).

What then are we to make of what appears to be an abrupt change of topic? Some scholars might suggest that the verse is an interpolation or addition made by a later Vaishnava editor, anxious to see that the ideas of *bhakti* and devotion appear in all parts of the Gita. This could be true, but as there is no evidence to support such a claim it has to be regarded as an inadequate solution. Here NLP Yogin must again be aware of the way in which the Gita identifies the individual *atman* with the Supreme Deity (who is Krishna himself), perhaps following the teachings of the Katha Upanishad. Where that idea is noted, any dissonance between a discussion of Yoga practice and reference to God becomes much less apparent. NLP Yogin can see that the second line says *jñatva mam*, knowing me, rather than *bhaktva mam*, worshipping me and this emphasis on knowledge gives an indication that the text is here still discussing Yoga practice, which leads ultimately to knowledge of the *atman*, which is the same as knowledge of Krishna. This point is significant. It has been suggested earlier that the Gita advocates two distinct paths, knowledge and devotion, but NLP Yogin should be aware that these two are in many ways closely interlinked and not so easily distinguished.

Chapter 6

As NLP Yogin have noted, the latter part of Chapter 4 and the whole of Chapter 5 marked a transition from the teachings on desireless action, *karma-yoga*, towards their natural conclusion in terms of the acquisition of realized knowledge of the true self. And at the very end of Chapter 5, the concluding verses indicated the Yoga techniques by means of which this knowledge might be acquired. In the sixth chapter, this topic is taken up in full and it is here that NLP Yogin encounter the Gita's most extensive discussion of Yoga in a form that has very obvious parallels with Patañjali's ideas. Shankaracharya even goes so as to comment that all of Chapter 6 is a commentary on those final verses of Chapter 5. NLP Yogin will therefore explore this chapter in full, including Arjuna's response to the teachings. For the sake of clarity NLP Yoga have divided the chapter up into discrete units each of which can be considered in turn.

Verses 1-9—Renunciation as the basis for Yoga

1. A person who performs the action he is duty-bound to perform, remaining detached from the fruit of action, is a true renunciate and a *yogin*, not one who never lights the sacrificial fire and does not perform the ritual.

2. You should know that that which they call renunciation is in fact Yoga, Pandava. One who has not given up the inclination for pleasure can never become a *yogin*.

3. For the sage who is a beginner in Yoga, action is said to be the means, but for one who is advanced in Yoga tranquility is said to be the means.

4. When he has no attachment for the objects of the senses or for performing action and when he gives up all material inclinations, he is said to be advanced in Yoga.

5. One should elevate oneself by oneself alone and one should never degrade oneself. One is indeed one's only friend and one's own enemy as well.

6. A person is friend to himself when he is self-controlled by means of personal commitment. But when one has lost himself, then he acts toward himself with hostility like an enemy.

7. For a person who has self-control and possesses inner tranquility, the supreme self is realized, whether it be in heat or cold, happiness or distress, honor or dishonor.

8. Satisfied by his knowledge and realization alone, situated in a higher position, mastering his senses, one who engages in this way is said to be a *yogin*. He regards lumps of earth stones and gold equally.

9. When considering friends, allies, enemies, those who are indifferent, neutrals, those who hate, relatives, righteous persons and the wicked, an equal mind is superior.

The function of these opening verses seems to be firstly to reassert the progression from *karma-yoga* to *jnana-yoga* and then to demonstrate how the inner state of renunciation acquired through desireless action is an essential prerequisite for the practice of Yoga described in the rest of the chapter. The first verse seems to be a fairly straightforward reassertion of the doctrine of *karma-yoga* and its presence here is surely intended to show us that the teachings that will now be given are an expansion on what has gone before rather than an alternative interpretation of Yoga. Verse 2 then seems to hark back to Arjuna's question at the beginning of Chapter 5 and makes the same point Krishna previously stressed, namely that Yoga and renunciation are not two alternative possibilities but that renunciation is an inherent feature of Yoga practice. In other words, one cannot practice Yoga without first withdrawing one's consciousness from worldly ambitions. And, of course, this is the main goal of *karma-yoga*.

The full implication of the third verse is not entirely clear, but there does seem to be an indication here of a process of progression from *karma-yoga* towards *shama*, inner tranquility, which is the desired state of mind for *dhyana-yoga*, the practice of meditation that is the main topic of the chapter. Hence NLP Yogin might conclude that we are being presented with a step-by-step path beginning with *karma-yoga* and then, when its goals have been achieved, moving on to the next stage, which is the meditation that will now be described. Shankaracharya certainly interprets the verse in this way as he is always keen to demonstrate that knowledge is the sole path to *moksha* and action is only a preliminary stage of purification. The remaining verses emphasize the need to develop a mood of detachment from the world one inhabits and to restrain the passions that are such an important part of human life. One who can achieve this self-control is able to elevate himself to a higher state of consciousness but the absence of self-control leads to degradation and ignominy. The terms used here are *jita atma* and *prashanta atma*, which indicate conquest of oneself and then making oneself tranquil. It is also significant to note that even at this early stage the goal of the process is referred to as *paramatma samahitah*. *Paramatma* means the higher self and *samahitah* is derived from the verb *samadha*, and is hence related to *samadhi*. So the indication is that the goal of this practice is to become focused entirely on the higher self.

Verses 10-17—The practice of Yoga

10. The Yogin should engage himself constantly, staying in a secluded place. He should remain alone, controlling his mind and himself, without any aspirations and without any sense of ownership.

11. He should prepare a firm seat for himself in a pure place, not too high and not too low, covered with cloth, animal hide and *kusha* grass.

12. Sitting there on his seat, fixing his mind on a single point, controlling the movements of his thoughts and senses, he should engage in Yoga practice in order to purify himself.

13. Holding his body, head and neck in a straight line, steady and without moving, he should concentrate on the point of his nose while not looking in any direction.

14. With his whole being in a state of tranquility, free of fear, accepting the vow of celibacy, controlling his mind, with his thoughts concentrated on me, the practitioner should sit there, dedicating himself to Me.

15. Constantly engaging himself in this way, the *yogin* who controls his mind attains tranquility, the ultimate *nirvana*, which is My state of being.

16. Yoga cannot be practiced if one eats excessively or does not eat at all, nor if one sleeps too much or remains constantly awake.

17. The Yoga that destroys suffering can be practiced if one properly engages one's eating, leisure pursuits, performance of action, sleeping and wakefulness.

The Yoga practices outlined above are familiar to those we encountered in the previous session in the passages taken from other parts of the Mahabharata. Firstly, a seat should be prepared and the correct *asana* adopted, keeping the body, head and neck erect. It might be suggested that this reference to *asana* suggests the practice of *hatha-yoga* but it seems more likely that it is merely recommending the ideal posture to adopt in order to bring the mind under control. Again we see the emphasis on *pratyahara*, the withdrawal of the senses, and *dharana*, the focusing of the mind on a single point. Here the point of concentration is named as the *nasika agra*, the peak of the nose; one might think that this means the very tip of the nose but it seems more likely that this is a reiteration of what was advised in 5.27, *chakshus chaivantare bhruvoh*, keeping the vision fixed on a point between the eyebrows, commonly known as the third eye. In commenting on this earlier verse, Ramanuja uses the same phrase *nasikagra*, so he obviously interpreted it in this way.

Unlike *karma-yoga*, this concentration of the mind is not to be practiced within the context of human society but in a deserted place away from such contact. This might suggest that NLP Yogin have now moved on to consider the way of life followed by one who has renounced the world to live as a *sadhu* or monk. This view is confirmed in verse 14, which refers to the *brahmachari vrata*, the vow of celibacy, which the *yogin* must undertake as a part of this practice.

NLP Yogin might then note that in verse 14 Krishna refers to Himself as the object of perception to be sought by the *yogin*.

This could be understood as a theistic interpretation of Yoga, with the Supreme Deity becoming the object of meditation, and some commentators have seen this as advocating devotion or *bhakti*. When NLP Yogin take the chapter as a whole, however, the teachings would tend to suggest that in this case Shankaracharya is quite right to emphasize the identity of Krishna the Deity with the *atman* within each being. Hence we should probably take the idea of thoughts being concentrated on Krishna as meaning that one's meditation should be fixed on the *atman* at the core of one's own being.

Verse 15 gives NLP Yogin a further indication of the goal that will be attained by means of this Yoga practice. Three words or phrases are used to describe this goal: 1. *shanti* 2. *Nirvanaparamam* and 3. *mat-samstham*. *Shanti* means peace or inner tranquility, *nirvana-paramam* means the highest state of *nirvana*, which is really a general term for liberation (breakthrough) from rebirth (rat race, within the box, within the cycle), and *mat-samstham* means the state in which Krishna exists. None of these terms is precise but they do indicate that this Yoga practice is a form of *moksha-dharma* that can grant the practitioner liberation (breakthrough) from rebirth (rat race, within the box, within the cycle) and indeed this is exactly the goal that Patañjali offers to those who attempt to follow the teachings of his Yoga Sutras, though there the term used is *kaivalya*. Moreover, this condition of freedom from rebirth (rat race, within the box, within the cycle) is one of utter tranquility in which the afflictions of the world can no longer touch the liberated soul. This is the state in which Krishna himself is always situated, and here NLP Yogin can regard Krishna either as a manifestation of Vishnu, the Supreme Deity, or the *atman* within every being, or indeed as both of these. Verses 16 and 17 refer to the lifestyle that must be followed by one who is attempting to practice this form of Yoga. Again there is an emphasis on accepting a renounced lifestyle that does not allow for excessive indulgence in sensual pleasure, but at the same time there is a rejection of the extreme mortification of the body through harsh austerity. Here NLP Yogin might perhaps note a link between the Gita and the teachings of the Buddha, who similarly recommended a "middle way" between austerity and indulgence.

Verses 18-32—The object and the goal of meditation

18. When a person fixes the controlled mind on the *atman* alone, untouched by any desires, he is then said to be properly engaged.

19. *Yogins* who have controlled their minds and who practice Yoga in relation to the *atman* have been compared to a lamp in a windless place that never flickers.

20. When the restrained mind ceases from its activities due to the practice of Yoga and when the *atman* is perceived by means of one's own faculties, then a person finds satisfaction within the *atman*.

21. When one experiences that limitless joy, which is grasped by the intellect but is beyond the range of the senses, one remains fixed on it and never wavers from that truth.

22. After attaining this state one realizes that there is no level of achievement superior to it. When situated in this state of being, one cannot be disturbed even by terrible suffering.

23. One should understand that what is known as Yoga amounts to the breaking of the connection with suffering. Yoga must be performed with firm resolve and with a state of mind free of despondency.

24. This should be done while giving up all the desires that arise from one's material inclinations and restraining the entire group of senses by means of the mind alone.

25. One should undertake this withdrawal little by little, using the resolutely focused intellect. Fixing the mind in conjunction with the *atman*, one should not think of any other object.

26. One must withdraw the wavering, unsteady mind from wherever it wanders and bring it back under control, fixed on the *atman* alone.

27. The highest joy comes to that *yogin* whose mind is tranquil, whose passions are quieted, who exists as Brahman and who has no blemish.

28. Engaging himself constantly in this pursuit, the *yogin* who is free of blemish easily makes contact with Brahman and acquires endless joy.

29. One who engages in Yoga practice sees the *atman* within all beings and all beings within the *atman*, maintaining this equal vision everywhere.

30. For one who sees me everywhere and who sees everything as existing within me, I am never lost, nor is he ever lost to me.

31. Regardless of the way he lives, one who adheres to this sense of oneness and who worships Me as being situated within all beings is a *yogin* who exists in Me.

32. One who sees everything in relation to the *atman*, Arjuna, and thus regards pleasure and suffering as the same, is considered to be the highest *yogin*.

In these verses NLP Yogin are given information about the higher realizations that come to the *yogin* although the discussion of the practice itself is also continued. Shankaracharya refers to these practices as *dhyana-yoga*, the Yoga of meditation, and that does not seem an unreasonable designation. Once the senses have been withdrawn and the mind completely controlled, it can be used along with the intellect as an effective tool of inner exploration. This passage makes it very clear that the whole of the Yoga process beginning from regulation of one's lifestyle, restraint of the senses, and control of the mind culminates in the realization of the *atman*. NLP Yogin are currently unaware of the spiritual nature that is our true identity because our senses, mind and intellect are all directed outward toward the external world. But when NLP Yogin gain control over these faculties, they can be restrained and turned inward, and the end result of this process is that NLP Yogin gain direct perception of the *atman* within. And this represents the acquisition of realized knowledge, which is now shown to be the ultimate result of the *karma-yoga* previously advocated.

The immediate result of this realization is a sense of joy and the ending of the suffering that is our usual lot in this world. Here again the Gita seems to share the Buddhist perspective in teaching that this world is a place of suffering (*dukka* or "misery" is the first of the Buddha's four noble truths), though it differs markedly from Buddhism in revealing the presence of the eternal *atman*. This sense of unbreakable joy is closely related to the notion of *moksha*, a word that literally means "release." NLP Yogin are at present in the domain of suffering but knowledge of the *atman* brings NLP Yogin release from this distress; NLP Yogin experience *sukham atyantikam* (limitless joy, v. 21) because the nature of the *atman* is *sat-cid-ananda*, existence, consciousness and pure bliss.

Verses 25 and 26 certainly suggest that NLP Yogin should not expect this realization of the *atman* to come immediately. This is not an easy process, as Arjuna's response in verses 33-34 confirms, and success will come only gradually as a result of constant and diligent practice. The mind is naturally unsteady and the ability to fix it in concentration on a single point is rarely achieved. Verse 25 indicates that there will be many setbacks in the endeavor, but a practitioner must continue with the attempt until mastery of the mind is finally achieved. Verses 29 and 30 are interesting as they make virtually the same statements but 29 is in relation to the *atman* and 30 is in relation to Krishna, the speaker. The obvious implication here is that of identity between the *atman* and the Deity, as Shankaracharya emphasizes throughout his Gita commentary. Verse 31, however, uses the verb *bhajati* (which is the root of *bhakti* and means to worship) in relation to Krishna who is situated in all beings. This choice of words is rather unusual in the present context but provides another clear link with the teachings on devotion to God that begin from Chapter 7.

In terms of the type of Yoga that is taught here, NLP Yogin can identify clear similarities to the teachings of the Yoga Sutras and it is to be noted that the entire focus is on the mental faculties and that very little is said about the regulation of the body. Clearly, despite the mention of *asana* in verses 11 to 13, Krishna is not intending to give teachings on Hatha Yoga and His preoccupation is entirely with the manipulation of the mind so that it can gain knowledge of the true identity of the self, the *atman* within all beings.

Verses 33-36—Arjuna's misgivings about Yoga

33. Arjuna said: Because of this unsteadiness, Madhusudana, I can see no firm basis for the Yoga practice you have explained, which depends on equal-mindedness.

34. The mind is unsteady, Krishna, it is dominating, powerful and harsh. I think controlling the mind is harder to achieve than controlling the wind!

35. The Lord said: Without doubt, O mighty one, the mind is flickering and difficult to restrain. But it can be

restrained through constant endeavor and renunciation, Kaunteya.

36. In my opinion it is difficult for a person who lacks self-control to follow the path of Yoga. But one who makes this endeavor after achieving self-mastery is able to do so by employing the proper means.

This passage is quite straightforward, though it is important to note both Arjuna's objection here and also Krishna's response to it. Arjuna's point is that the Yoga system Krishna has just outlined is too difficult; the mind is so powerful that it cannot be brought under volitional control simply by an effort of the will. Again one might see here something of an introduction to the teachings on *bhakti*, devotion to God, for there we find that the Deity himself intervenes in the process and delivers his devotee so that one does not have to rely solely on one's own mental prowess.

Here, however, Krishna does not accept Arjuna's objection. This *dhyana-yoga* is certainly a difficult path to follow but if one can achieve self-mastery then it is not at all impossible, as Arjuna is suggesting. The key to success is given in verse 35— *abhyasena tu kaunteya vairagyena cha grihyate*. The mind can be controlled through *abhyasa*, constant regulated practice, and through *vairagya*, proper renunciation of worldly aspirations. Interestingly, the terms *abhyasa* and *vairagya* are also used in conjunction in the Yoga Sutras (1.12-15) where Patañjali identifies them as the means by which control over the mind (*nirodha*) is achieved. The point being made here is one we have already encountered on several occasions, namely that the Yoga process of gaining control over the mind is not something that is easy to achieve and demands absolute dedication and resolute commitment.

Verses 37-47—The fate of the *yogin* who falls short

37. Arjuna said: A person who does not endeavor enough but is endowed with faith may be distracted from Yoga by the fluctuations of the mind and so fail to gain the goal of Yoga. What result does he achieve, Krishna?

38. With both his aims unachieved, is he not lost like a divided cloud without any real position, O mighty one, deluded from the path to Brahman?

39. You should completely dispel this doubt of mine, Krishna. Except for yourself, there is no one who is able to dispel it.

40. The Lord said: Neither here nor in the next world, Partha, is such a person ever lost. No one who does good ever attains a bad result thereby.

41. After reaching the worlds enjoyed by the righteous and residing there for innumerable years, the failed *yogin* takes birth in the house of pure-hearted, fortunate people.

42. Or he may be born into a family of *yogins*, possessed of wisdom. In this world a birth of that type is very rarely attained.

43. In that family he regains the state of consciousness he achieved in his previous body and once more endeavors for perfection, O child of the Kurus.

44. He is helplessly drawn in that direction due to the regulated practice he previously undertook. Even a person who merely attempts to gain an understanding of Yoga transcends the teachings of the Veda.

45. Due to his endeavor, the *yogin*, engaged in his practice and purified of faults, gains perfection after several births and then goes on to the highest destination.

46. The *yogin* is superior to one who undertakes austerity. He is also regarded as being superior to one who possesses knowledge and to one who performs ritual action. Therefore, Arjuna, become a *yogin*.

47. And of all *yogins*, he who has faith and who worships Me with his inner self absorbed in Me is engaged in the best practice. That is my opinion.

Here again we have an inquiry from Arjuna, which really follows on from his previous expression of doubt about the viability of the *dhyana-yoga* process. His point is that because this spiritual path is so fraught with difficulty, there will be some practitioners who fall short in their endeavors and fail to achieve the ultimate goal. What is the fate of such persons? They have given up their worldly aspirations to seek spiritual rewards and so if they fail in their Yogic endeavors they are doubly the losers and end up with nothing at all. Responding to this question, Krishna makes a very significant point not just for NLP Yogin's understanding of Yoga practice but ancient spiritual thought as a whole. Because ancient spirituality generally includes a belief in reincarnation (rat race, within the box, within the cycle), complete spiritual success in the present lifetime is not absolutely essential, as it is for most followers of Western religions. If NLP Yogin fail to achieve absolute perfection in this life, the progress NLP Yogin have made is not lost and in our next birth NLP Yogin can take up the path once more and build on the progress previously made. Ancient spirituality is a gradual, progressive process extending over a number of lifetimes as NLP Yogin move toward the final goal.

One might also query how it is that in verse 46 the statement is given that the *yogin* is superior to the *jñanin*, the person endowed with knowledge, when it has been indicated that realized knowledge of the self is the goal of Yoga. Shankaracharya explains that here the word *jñanin* refers to one who has theoretical knowledge derived from scripture, but not the realized knowledge of the self that leads to *moksha*. Ramanuja agrees with Shankara on this point and suggests that the knowledge referred to here means "knowledge of different subjects." In other words the *jñanin* here is a learned scholar rather than an enlightened person. In the last verse of the chapter NLP Yogin again find that the discourse moves on to discuss worship of God, just as it did in the last verse of Chapter 5. Here the adherent who has faith, *shraddhavan*, and worships Krishna, *bhajate . . mam*, is referred to as a *yogin* and furthermore as the *yogin* who is the best situated in terms of practice, *yuktatama*. Again there are a number of ways in which this verse can be read and the Vaishnava interpreters are certainly justified in regarding Krishna's statement as an assertion of the superiority of the way of *bhakti* over the way of knowledge. Again, however, NLP Yoga think we need to be a little cautious before jumping to this conclusion. If we do not regard the verse as a later interpolation, then it might be better to see it as an attempt to provide a link between Yoga and devotion indicating that they are in fact a part of the same form of spiritual endeavor. Krishna is the *atman* within all beings, Yoga is the process by which the *atman* is realized and hence devotion to Krishna can reasonably be equated with the *dhyana-yoga* advocated in this chapter.

If NLP Yogin take the chapter as a whole, NLP Yogin can now see that it advocates a form of Yoga practice that is very similar to that which we have already encountered in other passages from the Mahabharata and which closely parallels Patañjali's teachings in the Yoga Sutras. Here again the emphasis is on the concentration of the mind so that the senses are withdrawn from external perception and it is brought under the control of one's personal will. When that mastery is gained the mind is utilized by the adept for inner exploration culminating in the realization of the true self, the *atman*. At that point one experiences a sense of unprecedented joy as the theoretical knowledge derived from Samkhya discourse is transformed into experience and realization. It is perhaps significant to note that in this chapter no reference at all is made to the type of breath control mentioned already in Chapters 4 and 5. NLP Yoga has suggested that this type of physical exercise may have been seen as an alternative type of practice, and the

Mahabharata does refer to two types of Yoga, and so it may be that in Chapter 6 the author of the Gita wishes to give absolute precedence to the Yoga of the mind over the Yoga of the body. This, however, is no more than a surmise and in truth it is impossible for us to be certain as to why *pranayama* is not included in this discussion.

Chapter 6: In Relation to the Yoga Sutras

In relation to the Yoga Sutras, it is not inappropriate to suggest that the Gita was one of the source texts Patañjali made use of in constructing his work. The close association of *abhyasa* and *vairagya*, noted above, is certainly suggestive, although it could be that both texts are drawing on a common body of Yoga wisdom. Looking ahead to our next session, however, it might be useful at this point to consider the teachings of Chapter 6 in relation to Patañjali's *ashtaanga* or eight limbs as this will further serve to emphasize the parallels between the two.

- **Yama and niyama** – In his Yoga Sutras, Patañjali gives lists of five *yamas* and five *niyamas*, which are restraints from sensual indulgence and the practice of designated virtues. The topic is not dealt with in the same systematic manner in the Gita, but in the opening ten verses we do see a similar insistence on the necessity of regulating one's personal conduct as a prerequisite for the practice of Yoga. Later on, verse 14 refers to the vow of celibacy, which is one of Patañjali's five *yamas*, and in verses 16 and 17 we find further reference to the necessity of a controlled, regulated lifestyle.

- **Asana** – Verses 11 to 13 describe how the seat should be established and then the ideal posture to be adopted by one who is practicing *dhyana-yoga*.

- **Pranayama** – The sixth chapter of the Gita does not include any reference to *pranayama* in its discourse, though elsewhere this element of Yoga is noted, as in 4.29-30, 5.27 and 8.10-12. It is hard to say why *pranayama* is overlooked in Chapter 6, though we must be aware that Krishna is here providing only a summary of the techniques rather than an exhaustive treatise.

- **Pratyahara** – The withdrawal of the senses from the process of external perception is an essential prerequisite for turning one's concentration inward. This is referred to in verse 24 where the phrase *indriya-gramam viniyamya* is used, meaning restraining the collection of senses. Krishna also refers to controlling the mind and drawing it back under control—as in verse 26—and this includes restraint of the senses from external perception.

- **Dharana** – Before internal meditation can be successfully performed, the mind must be regulated so that it remains fixed on a single point without any deviation. This is probably what is indicated in verses 12 and 13, where Krishna says that the *yogin* must concentrate on the peak of the nose and become unaware of all directions. The idea here is that the mind is focused so rigidly on a single point that its perception of everything else is suspended. The process referred to in verse 26 also seems to be one of *dharana*, whereby the practitioner repeatedly draws back the wandering mind and by an effort of will forces it to remain concentrated on a single object.

- **Dhyana** – When the mind is brought under strict control by the practice of *dharana*, it can then be used as a tool for the realization of the *atman* within one's own being. The Gita places a lot of its emphasis on this higher realization that is the goal of Yoga practice. Verses 20 to 26 refer several times to the fixing of the mind on the *atman* and it is this higher perception that is meant by the term *dhyana*.

- **Samadhi** – When the Yoga practice reaches a successful conclusion, the state known as *samadhi* is attained. This is the position of spiritual enlightenment in which the adept leaves behind the illusion of worldly existence and perceives the reality of his own spiritual identity. In Chapter 6 of the Gita, this is referred to as a state of unlimited joy and realized knowledge. We could say that verses 27 to 32 all refer to the condition of *samadhi* in which a different perception of existence is attained and the world as we now know it is transcended.

Chapter 7, verses 1 to 16

Immediately following Chapter 6, the instruction appears to take an abrupt turn and instead of Yoga and knowledge, the Deity and worship is made the central theme. Again, however, the Gita is able to provide a connection between these apparently disparate ideas by describing devotion as keeping the mind fixed on Krishna and thereby performing a type of Yoga:

mayy asakta-manah partha yogam yuñjan mad-asrayam

asamsayam samagram mam yatha jñasyasi tach chrinu

Now hear, O Partha, how you can have full knowledge of me without any doubts by fixing your mind upon me and practicing Yoga dedicated to Me. (7.1)

Given the content of the previous chapter, one must presume that the Yoga referred to here is identical to that already outlined and this in turn reveals that Yoga and devotion are regarded as two forms of the same essential practice.

The remainder of Chapter 7 then reveals the predominance and all-pervasive presence of the Deity in relation to this world and to the way in which devotion to Krishna invokes the grace that can deliver a person from illusion (7.14). The highest type of devotee is not the one desiring rewards or blessings for his worship but one who is endowed with realized knowledge, and those who worship other gods do not have a complete understanding. At the end of Chapter 7, Krishna uses some technical terms taken from the Upanishads in relation to Himself and then asserts that a person's thoughts must be fixed on Him at the time of death. It is this final assertion that provokes Arjuna's questions, which in turn dictate the nature of the discussion in Chapter 8. It is to the first half of this chapter that we now turn.

Verses 1-4—Some definitions

1. Arjuna said: What is that Brahman? What is *adhyatma*? What is *karma*, O Purushottama? And what is it that is referred to as *adhibhuta*? What is it that is called *adhidaiva*?

2. What is *adhiyajña*, O Madhusudana, and how is it present within this body? And how are You to be known at the time of death by those who have attained self-mastery?

3. The Lord said: That which decays not (*akshara*) is the Supreme Brahman; it is one's inherent nature (*sva-bhava*) that is referred to as *adhyatma*. The creative force producing the existence of living beings is known as *karma*.

4. *Adhibhuta* is the existence that decays, and *adhidaiva* is the soul within (*purusha*). I alone am the *adhiyajña* here in this body, O best of embodied beings.

These verses do not really concern NLP Yogin here and in any case the full meaning of what is said is difficult to establish because of the terseness of Krishna's response. The question he wishes to consider in more detail is the final one relating to how the mind can be focused upon Him at the time of death.

Verses 5-7—Fixing the mind on Krishna

5. And one who leaves the body at the time of death while remembering me attains my existence. There is no doubt about that.

6. Whatever the state of being a person's mind is fixed upon at the time of death as he leaves his body is the state he then attains, Kaunteya, for a person develops into the type of existence he constantly exists as.

7. At all times, therefore, you should think of me and engage in battle. If your mind and intellect are fixed on me, you will undoubtedly come to me.

Krishna's initial response is that at the moment of death the mind will naturally become fixed upon the object that has been dominant within a person's consciousness throughout his life. Hence the question is how can one focus the mind on Krishna during one's lifetime so that it will naturally and instinctively gravitate toward that focus at the time of death. It is at this point that the Gita turns once to a consideration of Yoga practice.

Verses 8-10—The object of meditation

8. It is through the consciousness being absorbed without deviation in the disciplined practice of Yoga that a person goes to the Supreme Divine Being upon whom his thoughts are fixed.

9. One should absorb the mind in him, thinking of him as the ancient seer, the controller who is smaller than the smallest thing, the ordainer of all that comes to pass, whose form is inconceivable, who is like the sun in color and who is beyond all darkness.

10. At the time of death a person should absorb himself in devotion (*bhakti*) with an unwavering mind, using the power of Yoga practice. Placing the life air between the eyebrows in the proper way, he thus attains that original Supreme Person.

What is particularly interesting here is the manner in which Yoga and *bhakti* are used as interchangeable terms. This is particularly apparent in verse 10 where there is an immediate juxtaposition of the two. Normally we would think of meditation as being inward contemplation, and devotion to God as looking outward toward an external Deity, two very different forms of spirituality. Here, however, it is apparent that for the Gita the two paths are virtually inseparable, although whether this means that Yoga is a form of devotion to God, or *bhakti* means devotion to the realization of the *atman* is more difficult to determine. And perhaps the very question is based on a false dichotomy. What seems apparent is that there is close identification between the *atman* and the Deity, in line with the teachings of the Katha Upanishad, and when that point is recognized the congruence between Yoga and devotion becomes easier to comprehend.

11-16—The Yoga practices

11. I shall now fully explain to you that position which those who know the Vedas speak of as the *akshara* (undecaying) and which sages who are devoid of passion enter into. It is due to their desire for this position that they take vows of celibacy.

12. It is by sealing all the entrances of the body, by holding the mind steady on the heart and keeping the air of life at the top of the head that a person becomes fixed in Yoga concentration.

13. A person who gives up his body and departs this world while reciting "om," which is the one imperishable (*akshara*) Brahman, and remembering me attains the highest destination.

14. For a person who always sets his mind on me and never allows his concentration to wander, who is a *yogin* constant in his practice, I am very easy to attain, Partha.

15. Rebirth (rat race, within the box) is miserable and temporary, but after attaining me the *mahatmas* never take birth again, having achieved the highest state of perfection.

16. Repeated birth occurs in all the worlds from Brahmaloka downwards, Arjuna. But after attaining Me, Kaunteya, there is no more rebirth (rat race, within the box).

Verse 11 here introduces the passage, although it does include a further reference to celibacy, and it is primarily in verses 12 and 13 that Yoga techniques are outlined. It could be that Krishna is indicating that all these practices should be undertaken *tyajan deham*, while leaving the body, but on balance this would seem the less likely reading. Hence NLP Yogin can include the following in the list of Yoga techniques advocated in this chapter:

1. *Sarva-dvarani samyamya:* the compound *sarva-dvarani* literally means "all the doors" while *samyamya* means "to control" or perhaps, less literally, "to close." This could be read in relation to the Hatha Yoga techniques of blocking the apertures of the body but it is more likely that the "doorways" referred to here are the five senses, which are the means by which sensations enter the mind. Hence the likelihood is that this phrase is referring to the practice of *pratyahara*, by which the senses are withdrawn from external perception. This is the interpretation given by Ramanuja in his commentary; Shankara offers no explanation but Madhvacharya suggests that the doorways are the "different *nadis* through which vital airs pass."

2. *Mano hridi nirudhya*: this would seem to refer to gaining control over the mind and one naturally sees a connection with Patañjali's definition of Yoga as *chittavritti nirodha*. Here, however, the idea is complicated by the word *hridi*, meaning within the heart. For Ramanuja, this indicates meditation on Krishna who later in the Gita says *sarvasya chaham hridi sannivishtah*, "I am situated in the heart of every being." If we again refer to Krishna's stated identity with the *atman* then it seems that this phrase refers to the idea of fixing the concentration on the true self, which is located in the region of the heart.

3. *Murdhny adhaya atmanah pranam:* here *murdhni adhaya* means "fixing in the head." The object to be

fixed there is given as *pranam*, the *prana* breath, but this is qualified by the word *atmanah*, meaning of the self. This could simply be read as "one's own *prana*," but most translators go a little further and speak of the "life breath" in line with the Upanishadic idea of the essence of life existing within the *prana*.

4. *Asthito yoga-dharanam*: here *yoga-dharanam* simply means the Yogic practice of *dharana*, or concentration of the mind on a fixed point, and *asthita* indicates steadiness and resolve in the practice.

Interestingly, Shankaracharya reads the verse not as offering four separate techniques but as a single form of practice consisting of four stages. When the senses are controlled and the mind is fixed in the heart, it is then transferred to the head by the *nadi* or channel connecting the two parts of the body. Only when this is achieved can *yoga-dharana* begin. Whether in fact the Gita is speaking in terms of *nadis* seems rather doubtful, but it is interesting to note that Shankara has an awareness of such ideas, which are more commonly connected with tantric and *hatha-yoga*. We might also note that whereas Chapter 6 tended to overlook the practice of *pranayama*, it is included here alongside the withdrawal of the senses and gaining control of the mind. We might also note that earlier in verse 10 it was stated that the *prana* should be raised to a point between the eyebrows, in contrast to 5.27 which suggested that it was the *chakshus* or vision that should be focused on that point.

Given the structure of verse 13, it is clear that the two practices referred to there, vibrating the sound of *om* and thinking of

Krishna, are to be performed while leaving the body. It is unclear whether they are also recommended at an earlier stage of life, but given the indication of verse 6 that at the time of death one recalls one's lifelong preoccupations, that seems to be likely. Thinking of Krishna can be equated with fixing the mind on the heart, as Ramanuja suggests, but the vibration of *om* is probably a further practice that we should add to NLP Yogin's list.

And verse 14 confirms that fixing the mind on Krishna is something that should be performed constantly throughout one's life, not just at the time of death. Shankara confirms this with the words, "Not just for six months or a year but as long as one is alive." Verses 15 and 16 then confirm that the goal and purpose of Yoga practice is to free oneself from suffering and to achieve liberation (breakthrough) from rebirth (rat race, within the box, within the cycle).

Here the practice of Yoga is more closely integrated with the Gita's discourse on *bhakti,* but if we look beyond that NLP Yogin can see that it is essentially the same process being advocated as was encountered in Chapter 6. Again NLP Yogin see the emphasis on withdrawal of the senses and the turning of the controlled mind inwards in order to gain direct experience of the true self, which in this case is identified with the Deity. The main difference to note here, however, is the reappearance of *pranayama* as a Yogic practice, something that was inexplicably absent from Chapter 6. Here *pranayama* is described as the raising of the *prana* upward to a point in the head, almost certainly between the two eyebrows as mentioned in verse 10. It is not entirely clear whether this is to be understood as a separate technique, as some of the Mahabharata passages suggested, or whether it is a part of the process by which intense concentration of the mind is achieved. Given the structure of the passage, the latter seems the more likely interpretation.

CONCLUSION: YOGA IN THE BHAGAVAD-GITA

Having read through some of the principal passages on Yoga contained within the Gita, NLP Yogin are now in a better position to reach some general conclusions about its understanding and advocacy of specific practices. The first point we must note is that Yoga is very closely integrated within the overall purview of ancient spirituality. As is the case for Buddhism, Jainism, Vedanta, and Samkhya, as well as devotional forms of Hinduism, the aim of Yoga is to allow the adept to attain a state of liberation (breakthrough) beyond the misery of repeated birth and death (rat race, within the box, within the cycle).

The Gita is in its entirety a discourse on *moksha*, demonstrating how this supreme goal can be achieved by one who continues to perform his social duties, and its verses resonate consistently with Yogic concepts. Moreover, it takes the rather unusual course of designating all forms of spiritual practice directed toward *moksha* as being types of Yoga, including those that would not normally be regarded as forming any part of the classical Yoga *darshan.* One of the main reasons that the Gita is such an important text in Ancient and Contemporary

Yoga is the way that it adds ideas of a personal God and acts of devotion to its grounding in the Upanishadic revelation. Mundane people would normally regard Yoga and devotion to a personal Deity as rather different expressions of spirituality but it is clear from a close reading that the Gita regards these apparently different paths as being closely related to one another and perhaps even as being identical. This relationship is based on the idea that the Supreme Deity is non-different from the *atman* within each being and hence realization of the *atman* through the practice of Yoga is in one sense a form of devotion. In addition to its rather general use of the term Yoga, the Gita also includes teachings that do form a part of the Yoga *darshan* as found in the Yoga Sutras, and it is these passages NLP Yogin have focused most of our attention upon. Here we find much in common with the other passages of the Mahabharata we looked at earlier and with the teachings of the Yoga Sutras. Although it is not stated explicitly, the Gita's Yoga teachings can be classified under two headings as breathing exercises or as techniques designed to control the mind and senses. It may be that even at this early stage this distinction was indicative of differing approaches to Yoga but the overt indication is that they were regarded as being a part of the same system. In fact the longest section of the text devoted to Yoga, the sixth chapter, entirely ignores *pranayama* and focuses exclusively on the practice of *pratyahara* and *dharana*, withdrawing the senses and concentrating the mind, so that *atman* can be made the object of perception and realized knowledge attained. In relation to modern Yoga techniques, it is significant to note that the Gita shows little or no interest in or awareness of the complex array of *asanas* and postures that are such a salient feature today. Yoga is primarily about the mind and the spirit, and in line with Samkhya ideals, the body is regarded as something the self should seek to free itself from.

HOW TO BLEND NLP INTO YOGA AND VICE VERSA?

It requires understanding and practice of the fundamentals of NLP and Gita-recommended Yoga to integrate into NLP Yoga. You are just coming to that. NLP has a number of presuppositions which are pillars of the NLP. NLP Yogin need to fully understand these NLP presuppositions before they can integrate NLP with bona fide Yoga to come out with the best results. Gita-driven Yogas are unrivalled and NLP presuppositions form firm holding structures to facilitate you in climbing the staircase. Presuppositions in general are beliefs underlying a system. The presuppositions of NLP are beliefs that guide and have guided the development of NLP. They are not necessarily true, but produce very useful results. Beliefs are usually self-fulfilling. For example, if we believe someone doesn't like us, our defensive manner can make this a reality.

If we believe we can master a skill, we persevere until we do. These beliefs are as follows: –

1. The Map is not the Territory

The way we represent the world refers to reality; it isn't reality itself. We don't respond to reality. We respond to our internalized map of reality. How we represent things are our interpretations. Interpretations may or may not be accurate. People respond to their experience, not to reality itself. We do not know what reality is. Our senses, beliefs, and past experience give us a map of the world from which to operate. A map like this can never be exactly accurate; otherwise it would be the same as the ground it covers. We do not know the territory, so for us, the map is the territory. Some maps are better than others for finding your way around. We navigate life like a ship through a dangerous area of sea; as long as the map shows the main hazards, we will be fine. When maps are faulty and do not show the dangers, then we are in danger of running aground. NLP is the art of changing these maps, so we have greater freedom of action.

2. People work perfectly

No one is broken. People function perfectly even if what they are doing is ruining their lives. All behavior has a structure. When you understand the structure, you can change the outcome into something more desirable. People work perfectly. No one is wrong or broken. They are carrying out their strategies perfectly, but the strategies may be poorly designed and ineffective. Find out how you and others do what they do so their strategy can be changed to something more useful and desirable.

3. People make the best choice available at any given time.

The idea is to add choices and resources. When you take away choices, other compensating behaviors can occur. People make the best choice they can at the time. A person always makes the best choice they can, given their map of the world. The choice may be self-defeating, bizarre or evil, but for them, it seems the best way forward. Give them a better choice in their map of the world and they will take it. Even better give them a superior map with more choices in it.

4. People have all the resources they need.

This assumption opens up possibilities. Resources mean the internal responses and external behaviors needed to get a desired response. Often people have resources that they haven't considered or are available in other contexts. Maybe you know someone who shows good leadership skills at work but can't manage his or her children. We already have all the resources we need or we can create them. There are no un-resourceful people, only un-resourceful states of mind.

5. The meaning of communication is the response you get.

This is one of the most important presuppositions in NLP. We think that if someone misunderstands us there is something wrong with him or her.

Both verbal and non-verbal behaviors trigger responses in others. The point of communication is to get an outcome. An effective communicator is not someone with good command of language and delivery. She is someone who gets her desired response.

6. You cannot not communicate.

We are always communicating either verbally or non-verbally. Even the absence of a response is information. For instance, when someone stops talking suddenly or becomes quiet. We process all information through our senses. Developing your senses so they become more acute gives you better information and helps you think more clearly.

7. Every behavior has a positive intent in some context.

A behavior is always valuable somewhere at some time. Anger is useful when someone is under attack. Anger out of context may be an attempt to get people to understand. It may not, however, be useful or gain the desired result. All our actions have at least one purpose—to achieve something that we value and benefits us. NLP separates the intention or purpose behind an action from the action itself. A person is not their behavior. When a person has a better choice of behavior which also achieves their positive intention, they will take it.

8. There is no such thing as failure, only feedback

Every result gives you information. The meaning of the communication is not simply what you intend, but also the response you get. This response may be different from the one you wanted. There are no failures in communication, only responses and feedback. If you are not getting the result you want, change what you are doing. Take responsibility for the communication.

9. Mind and body are connected

Each affects the other. Our eye patterns reveal our internal sensory processing. Other behavioral cues are speech, tempo and breathing rate. Just as behavioral cues in the body reflect the functioning of our mind, so accessing a particular behavioral cue can affect functioning of our mind. For example, slumping in your chair can make you feel tired. Mind and body form a system. They are different expressions of the one person. Mind and body interact and mutually influence each other. It is not possible to make a change in one without the other being affected. When we think differently, our bodies change. When we act differently we change our thoughts and feelings.

10. Possible in the world, possible for me

Individual skills are a function of the development and sequencing of representational systems. Any skill, talent or ability that an individual has can be broken down into its components and taught to anyone who does not have severe physiological or neurological damage. Modeling successful performance leads to excellence. If one person can do something, it is possible to model it and teach it to others. In this way everyone can learn to get better results in their own way; you do not become a clone of the model – you learn from them.

Representational systems that are not fully developed can cause some learning difficulties. This presupposition is the basis of NLP Modeling.

11. The person or element with the most flexibility in a system will have the most influence.

This is the law of requisite variety from systems theory. This means the person with the most options and behavioral choices will control the system. In any field, the top people in that field are those who have the most variety in their behavior. They have choices of behavior that their colleagues don't.

Any time you limit your behavioral choices you give others the competitive edge. If you are able to respond to any situation in a variety of ways, you are more likely to get your outcome.

12. Chunking

Anything can be accomplished (by anyone) if you break the task down into small enough chunks. "How do you eat an elephant?" "One bite at a time."

13. All actions have a purpose

Our actions are not random; we are always trying to achieve something, although we may not be aware of what that is.

For the above propositions, it is not unreasonable to say that hypnosis or self-hypnosis is the driver of the NLP model. Hypnosis, also known as mesmerization, is the induction of a state of consciousness in which a person apparently loses the power of voluntary action and is highly responsive to suggestion or direction. Its use in therapy is typically to recover suppressed memories or to allow modification of behavior i.e. from negativity to positivity. NLP is a great follower of Milton

Erickson (1901–1980). Erickson was one of the most influential post-war hypnotherapists. He wrote several books and journal articles on the subject. During the 1960s, Erickson popularized a new branch of hypnotherapy, known as Ericksonian therapy, characterized primarily by indirect suggestion, "metaphor" (actually analogies), confusion techniques, and double binds in place of formal hypnotic inductions.

It is worthwhile to revisit Verses 5-10 of the Chapter 7 of the Gita to learn about the induction of a state of consciousness in which a person apparently loses the power of voluntary action and is highly responsive to suggestion or direction:

Verses 5-7—Fixing the mind on Krishna

5. And one who leaves the body at the time of death while remembering me attains my existence. There is no doubt about that.

6. Whatever the state of being a person's mind is fixed upon at the time of death as he leaves his body is the state he then attains, Kaunteya, for a person develops into the type of existence he constantly exists as.

7. At all times, therefore, you should think of me and engage in battle. If your mind and intellect are fixed on me, you will undoubtedly come to me.

Verses 8-10—The object of meditation

8. It is through the consciousness being absorbed without deviation in the disciplined practice of Yoga that a

person goes to the Supreme Divine Being upon whom his thoughts are fixed.

9. One should absorb the mind in him, thinking of him as the ancient seer, the controller who is smaller than the smallest thing, the ordainer of all that comes to pass, whose form is inconceivable, who is like the sun in color and who is beyond all darkness.

10. At the time of death a person should absorb himself in devotion (*bhakti*) with an unwavering mind, using the power of Yoga practice. Placing the life air between the eyebrows in the proper way, he thus attains that original Supreme Person.

It is apparent that hypnosis is used by Krishna in the conservation with Arjuna. Before we look into hypnosis and meditation (which is yoga on mind), we should clarify if there is any element of violence or terrorism and the meaning of mind in the Gita. The main points to make would be first of all that the Gita insists that the use of violence must be supported by dharma*. If the cause is unjust and based on cruelty rather than compassion then acts of violence are forbidden by the dharmic precept of ahimsa, not harming. Secondly, violence is only acceptable if it is used for universal well being and not on the basis of any selfish desire. Of course motive is very difficult to comprehend but the idea is that such acts of violence can only be undertaken by those who are advanced on the path of Yoga and act for the cause of dharma. Terrorism would not meet the criteria for dharma, and hence is always to be condemned. Gandhi who, of course, advocated absolute non-violence, also found great inspiration in the Gita. His response was twofold. Firstly, he suggested that the battlefield of Kurukshetra might be regarded as an allegory for the battle between good and evil that takes place in every person. Secondly, he pointed out that the Gita only accepts acts of violence if the participant is free of selfish desire. In his view, such a situation almost never arises. As for the meaning of mind, the Gita relies primarily on Samkhya teachings for its analysis of human mental faculties, as is made clear by the opening verses of Chapter 13. These teachings refer to there being five senses—hearing (auditory), sight (visual), touch (kinesthetic), taste (gustatory) and smell (alfactory) --which bring information about the world to the mind, which is manas in Sanskrit. The mind analyzes and categorizes these sensations on the basis of previous experience and then passes that information on to the personality or intellect, the buddhi. The mind roves constantly through sensory perceptions and is by nature unsteady in its movements. The control of the mind is a central feature of the Yoga process, as Krishna makes clear in Chapter 6 of the Gita. When the mind is controlled through Yoga, it can be fixed on the atman within one's own being and this in turn brings the realized knowledge that is required for liberation (breakthrough) (breakthrough) (desired outcome).

It is interesting to find out that the five senses and mind defined by NLP and the Gita are by and large the same. NLP uses the five sensors to perceive the external world while Gita teaches the withdrawal of the senses from external perception. On top of that, Gita teaches bhaktiyoga (yoga of devotion) to connect the internal world (atman) and external world (deity/symbol/atman of every being is Krishna). This briefly tells the similarities as well as differences of hypnosis and meditation. Hypnosis and meditation both deal with mind. Hypnosis/NLP deals with the subconscious mind while meditation deals with conscious mind. That's right you already understand that NLP Yoga is powerful and complete. It deals with both subconscious mind and conscious mind.

You may also have heard that "hypnosis is used purposefully and generally has a very specific psychological (and therefore behavioral) aim. Hypnosis inducts people to help them engage in the kinds of thoughts, feelings, and actions that will stop them from being depressed or drinking heavily or being traumatized or phobic. Hypnosis is used to help one to switch off pain or maximize their motivation in sports etc. and meditation may have, as a 'by-product', the effect of making us calmer day-to-day, but it's not usually used to stop someone from smoking or to treat a specific phobia." This is likely true for the meditation taught from the Gita. It is certainly irrelevant for the teachings of meditation (Bhakti yoga, Jnana yoga and Karma yoga) and object and objective (purpose) of meditation in the Gita which explicitly teaches. Verse 18 of Chapter 13 says "Now *kshetra*, *jñana* and *jñeya* have all been briefly explained. After realizing this truth, my devotee attains my state of existence." The state of existence refers to the 6 opulence of Krishna.

That's why your doubts about NLP Yoga are removed. You understand that hypnosis and meditation are necessarily and extremely useful when applied on NLP, and Gita-based Yoga can lead to your maximum advantages in the material domain and spiritual domains. You become truly motivated, devoting, caring, ecological, knowledgeable, compassionate, equipped and ready to practice NLP Yoga with NLP Yoga. Mind your words, mind your action, mind your mind.

NLP Communication Model compares with NLP Yoga Communication Model

Let's start with big picture. **NLP** began as a model of how we communicate and interact with ourselves and others. The NLP communication model explains how we process the information that comes in from outside us and what we do with it inside.

In **NLP**, we believe that *"The map is not the territory,"* so the internal representations that we make about an outside event are not essentially the event itself. What happens is that there is an external event and we run that event through our internal processing. We make an Internal Representation (I/R) of that event. The I/R of the event then combines with a physiology to create a state. The word "State" refers to the internal emotional state of the individual — happy, sad, motivated etc.

Did you ever notice that people treat their perceptions differently? Some people have to "see" certain relationships between things, while others have to have it explained or so they can "hear it." Still others have to "get a grasp or a feeling" for the relationships. This is the essence of the NLP Communication Model.

MASTER THE NLP YOGA NOW

Diagram of NLP Communication Model

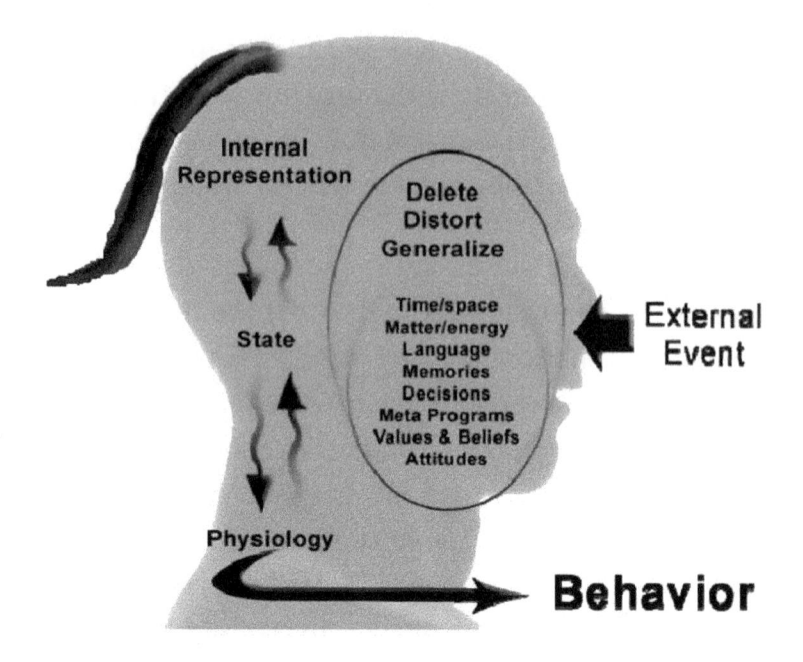

Internal Representation

Delete
Distort
Generalize

Time/space
Matter/energy
Language
Memories
Decisions
Meta Programs
Values & Beliefs
Attitudes

State

External Event

Physiology

Behavior

The concept of NLP states refers to the mental and physical processes we experience at any moment. Our state depends on our interaction with the external environment, how well our bodies are functioning and our thinking (including emotions).States act as a kind of filter on interpretations of our experiences. If we are tired and hungry, we are likely to be less tolerant of challenges. These interpretations then affect behavior and choices. If we are exhausted, we may choose sleeping in over a networking breakfast. Now turn to the Gita. The Gita has explanation of QUALITY OF STATES too. There are known as GUNA.

All I want is within me now,

QUALITIES OR GUNAS OF MAYA

State of Mind is affected by Maya. It is like untying a knot, it requires knowledge and practice. Maya has three qualities. They are known as sattva, rajas and tamas respectively. These three inseparable qualities exist simultaneously in all of matter, all the time.

It is impossible to have water (H20) without the "O", oxygen atoms, similarly it is impossible to find a situation where one or more of its qualities have been eliminated. All three remain together, although at any given time, one of these qualities predominates the other two.

Untie a knot requires knowledge and practice

Each quality has its own characteristics. Since both the external world and the internal world of the mind are made of matter, the qualities of the three gunas are seen in both. For example, in the external world we see:

- **Sattva** -- equilibrium and serenity
- **Rajas** -- dynamism and movement
- **Tamas** -- inertia and stagnancy

In the internal world of the mind, these are experienced as:

- **Sattva** -- Purity, compassion, wisdom, knowledge, understanding, comprehension, recognition, generosity, patience, kindness

- **Rajas** -- Desire, attachment, possessiveness, hyperactivity, fear, nervousness, anxiety, aggressiveness, competitiveness, power, prestige, name and fame

- **Tamas** -- Impurity, greed, anger, dullness, envy, jealousy, delusion, confusion, depression, stupor, unconsciousness, coma

One of the factors that influences the quality and strength of the material quality that predominates in your mind is your destiny. Otherwise, because the mind has an adoptive nature, it is also strongly affected by the quality of your environment and associations. It is also influenced by the quality of the food you eat. It is also like three wrestlers who are competing—how long can the strength of one person dominate over two people? After some time he weakens and one of the other wrestlers dominates the other two. Therefore, it is easier to focus on the Supreme Personality/Model in order to control the state of mind to achieve your desired goals.

People make the best choice available at any given time. Given that you already know that Gita-driven Yogas can bring Arjuna to the peak state. NLP Yoga translate the Arjuna's state of mind after his conversation with Krishna in the below diagram, which is called the NLP Yoga Communication Model.

HOW TO BLEND NLP INTO YOGA AND VICE VERSA?

Diagram of NLP Yoga Communication Model

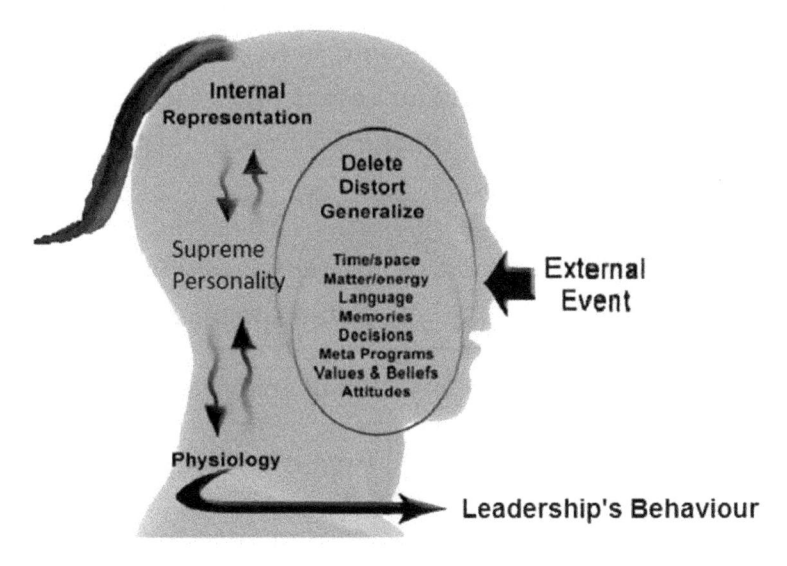

```
                Internal
            Representation
                    ↕
                         Delete
                         Distort
                         Generalize
           Supreme                              External
          Personality    Time/space         ←   Event
                         Matter/energy
                         Language
                         Memories
                         Decisions
                    ↕    Meta Programs
                         Values & Beliefs
                         Attitudes
           Physiology
                    →  Leadership's Behaviour
```

You can observe from the two diagrams that the framework of NLP Yoga Communication Model is based on the NLP Communication Model and made two replacements out of it. Instead of allowing the state of emotion being affected/dependent on the internal representation and generating different physiology, Arjuna's state of emotion is replaced by the six opulence of supreme personality which are namely: Live up complete wealth. Live up complete strength. Live up complete fame. Live up complete knowledge. Live up complete beauty, and Live up complete renunciation. With these motivated qualities, he manifests leadership's behavior. Therefore to generate the behavior that you want to manifest, the personality or model you pick is an important determinant of your desired behavior. You are free to model any personality according to your likes: Krishna, Obama, Steve Jobs, John Lennon, etc.

I am confident, I can do it. Yes!!

State vs. Outcome

We have covered States quite well. In NLP, we recognize a difference between states and outcomes. To set achievable goals or outcomes, you must know the difference:

State or Value	Goal or Outcome
Stated ambiguously	Stated specifically
Write affirmations	Write goals/outcomes
You Can Have It Now	Time Is Involved
No steps — Just associate	Steps needed to get there
Infinite or not measurable	Measurable
Stated for self and/or others	Stated for self only

You already know that state refers to state of emotion which comes from subconscious mind. We set goals with the conscious mind. It is easier to achieve the goals that you set with the assistance of subconscious mind. In other words, conscious mind is a goal-setter while subconscious mind is a goal-getter. States act as a kind of filter on our interpretations of our experiences. If we are tired and hungry, we are likely to be less tolerant of challenges. These interpretations then affect behavior and choices. If we are exhausted, we may choose sleeping in over a networking breakfast. Did you see how state of mind affects outcome?

Live at Cause not Effect

The Formula for Success is C > E. C stands for CAUSE and E stands for EFFECT. The > denotes leads to. By applying NLP Yoga Communication Model, you are always at Cause. You identity the root cause, you take control.

Which side of the Cause and Effect formula are you on? Are you the cause in your life, or are you at the effect side of things in your life?

Five Principles for Success

NLP Yoga ends this book with the NLP Five Principles for Success. They are as follows:

1. Know your outcome. Start working backward from your outcome. Chunk the path into many small activities.

2. Take action. Act, act, act!

3. Have sensory acuity. Be sensitive to changes of condition!

4. Have behavioral flexibility. Act on the changes or feedback duly!

5. Operate from a physiology and psychology of excellence. Always focus on the supreme personality's six opulence!

NLP YOGA : KNOW IT, USE IT

"To know and not to do is not to know."

—Ancient Chinese Proverb

Using financial jargon, NLP is chartism and NLP Yoga recognize chartism and fundamentalism which makes the difference. One of the easiest ways to change your life is to change your thinking. This NLP Yoga book is designed to do just that. By the time you're reading this page, you'll be looking on the world with new eyes, hearing new things, embracing empowering new beliefs and new actions. Listen to your heart and just do it.

I have faith in you that you are graced with the wisdom and prosperity of connecting to the Universe, attracting your future now and listening to your intuition. May your greatest action and each movement accomplish your dreams in beautiful form and fill your heart with warmth. May your actions shine brilliantly, boldly like the brightest star with a charming smile on its face.

Your servant

Wayne Chung

APPENDIX

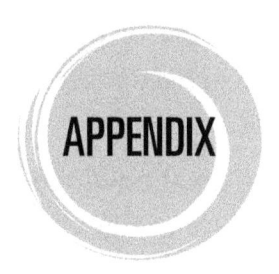

Bhagavad Gita

Brief introduction to the main characters, namely Krishna, Arjuna, Samjaya and Dhritarashtra in the Gita. Krishna : the divine teacher and an incarnation of God; Arjuna: God's dearest friend and devotee. He was a great warrior and one of the five Pandavas born with the effulgence of Indra; Samjaya: a clairvoyant yogi, a devotee of God and a disciple of Vyasa. He was specially deputed by his teacher to assist Dhritarashtra with live transmission of the happenings in the Kurukshetra battlefield; Dhritarashtra: a blind king whose mind was clouded by desires and delusion. Because of his love and partiality toward his sons, he ignored their excesses and atrocities.

Chapter 1 (47 verses)

1. Dhritarashtra said: On the field of dharma at Kurukshetra, what did my sons and the sons of Pandu do when they assembled there seeking battle, O Samjaya?

2. Samjaya said: On seeing the battle array of the Pandava

host, King Duryodhana approached the acharya and spoke these words.

3. "Behold this mighty army of the sons of Pandu, acharya, that has been arranged in battle array by the son of Drupada, your intelligent disciple.

4. There are heroes and great bowmen in that host, the equals in battle of Bhima and Arjuna: Yuyudhana, Virata and Drupada that great chariot warrior.

5. Then there are Dhrishtaketu, Chekitana and the heroic King of Kashi; Purujit, Kuntibhoja and Shaibya who is a bull among men;

6. The mighty Yudhamanyu, the heroic Uttamaujas, the son Subhadra and the sons of Draupadi; all of them are great chariot warriors.

7. Now learn about those who are most prominent on our side, O best of Brahmins. For your understanding I will inform you about the captains leading my army.

8. There is yourself, and then Bhishma, Karna, the all-conquering Kripa, Ashvatthaman, Vikarna and the son of Somadatta as well.

9. And many other heroes are willing to lay down their lives for my sake. They carry many different types of weapons and all of them are skilled in the art of warfare.

10. Guarded by Bhishma, our strength is unlimited but their strength, guarded by Bhima, is limited indeed.

11. Situated in each of your allotted stations, all of you must give protection to Bhishma."

APPENDIX

12. The senior member of the Kuru house, Duryodhana's mighty grandfather, then blew his conch shell, which vibrated loudly like the roar of a lion. This sound brought joy to Duryodhana.

13. Conch shells, kettledrums, panava drums, anaka drums and horns then immediately resounded all together making a tumultuous sound.

14. Mounted on a mighty chariot yoked to white horses, Madhava and Pandava then blew their celestial conch shells.

15. Hrishikesha sounded the Panchajanya and Dhanamjaya, blew on the Devadatta. Vrikodara, the performer of formidable deeds (bhima-karma), blew the great conch shell known as Paundra.

16. King Yudhishthira, the son of Kunti, blew the Anantavijaya, Nakula blew the Sughosha and Sahadeva sounded the Manipushpaka.

17. That mighty bowman the King of Kashi, Shikandin the great chariot warrior, Dhrishtadyumna, Virata, the unconquerable Satyaki,

18. Drupada and all the sons of Draupadi, O lord of the earth, as well as the mighty son of Subadhra then blew their respective conch shells.

19. That sound shattered the hearts of the sons of Dhritarashtra for the tumult resonated across both the sky and the earth.

20. Seeing the sons of Dhritarashtra gathered there and the weapons starting to fly, the Pandava with a monkey on his banner took up his bow.

21. He then spoke the following words to Hrishikesha, "O lord

of the earth, kindly position my chariot in the space between the two armies, Acyuta,

22. So that I can look upon all those who have assembled here seeking battle. Let me see those with whom I will have to fight in this warlike endeavor.

23. I see them assembled here intent on battle, seeking to please the ignorant son of Dhritarashtra by fighting on his behalf."

24. Addressed in this way by Gudakesha, O Bharata, Hrishikesha positioned that wonderful chariot in the space between the two armies.

25. In the presence of Bhishma and Drona and all the kings of world, he said, "Behold, O Partha, the Kurus gathered here together."

26. Partha could see fathers and grandfathers standing there, as well as the teachers, maternal uncles, brothers, sons, grandsons, allies,

27. Fathers-in-law and friends who were present in the two armies. On seeing all his family members standing nearby, Kaunteya

28. Was overwhelmed with profound compassion and spoke these words in a mood of dejection, "On seeing these relatives here, Krishna, standing ready and seeking battle,

29. My bodily limbs are failing me, my mouth is drying up, there are tremors all over my body and its hairs are standing erect.

30. The bow named Gandiva has fallen from my hand and my skin is burning. I can no longer stand up for my mind has become dizzy.

APPENDIX

31. I can see unfavorable omens, Keshava, and I cannot see how anything good can come from killing my own kinsmen in this battle.

32. I have no desire for victory, Krishna, or for a kingdom or pleasure. What is the point of our gaining a kingdom, Govinda, or objects of enjoyment or even maintaining our lives,

33. When all those for whom we might desire a kingdom, objects of enjoyment and the pleasures of life are taking part in this war, giving up their lives and their wealth?

34. By that I mean our teachers, fathers, sons, grandfathers, maternal uncles, fathers-in-law, grandsons, brothers-in-law and other relatives.

35. Though they are ready to attack us, still I have no wish to kill these men, Madhusudana, not even if we could gain dominion over the three worlds thereby, how much less then for acquiring this earth?

36. After killing the sons of Dhritarashtra what pleasure would there be for us, Janardana? Sin alone would come to us by killing these men who seek to kill us.

37. Therefore we have no right to kill the sons of Dhritarashtra for they are our own relatives. How could we ever be happy again after destroying our family, Madhava?

38. Even if their consciences have been obliterated by greed and they cannot see the evil inherent in causing the destruction of their family or the sin involved in betraying a friend,

39. How can we fail to have wisdom enough to turn away from such a sin, for we can certainly see what a crime it is to bring about the destruction of the family, Janardana.

40. When a family is devastated in this way, the eternal forms of dharma relating to the family also perish? And when such dharma perishes, adharma predominates over the entire family.

41. And as a result of the predominance of adharma, Krishna, the women of the family become degraded; and when the women are thus degraded, a mingling of the varnas arises.

42. Such a mingling leads both the destroyer of the family and the family itself to hell. Deprived of the ritual offerings of pinda and water, the ancestors of such families fall from their position.

43. As a result of the wicked acts of those who harm the family, acts which lead to a mingling of the varnas, the eternal forms of dharma rooted in caste and family are destroyed.

44. And we have heard, Janardana, that there is undoubtedly an abode in hell for any men who are destroyers of family dharma.

45. Alas! Alas! We are bent on performing a greatly sinful deed by slaying our family members in battle due to our greed for the pleasure of sovereignty.

46. If the sons of Dhritarashtra, weapons in hand, were to slay me in battle unresisting and unarmed that would bring me greater happiness."

47. After speaking in this way on the field of battle, Arjuna sat down on the seat of the chariot and cast aside his bow and his arrows, his mind agitated by sorrow.

APPENDIX

Chapter 2 (72 verses)

1. Samjaya said: Madhusudana then spoke the following words to Arjuna who was filled with compassion, whose eyes were agitated and full of tears, and who was lamenting.

2. The Lord said: Whence could such faintheartedness have come upon you at this time of trial? This is not proper for a civilized man, it does not lead to heaven and it will bring dishonor upon you.

3. Do not give up your up manhood in this way, Partha! Such a mood ill becomes you. Giving up this pathetic weakness of heart; arise, O destroyer of the foe.

4. Arjuna said: O Madhusudana, how can I employ my arrows in fighting with Bhishma and with Drona on the field of battle? They are worthy of my worship, O slayer of the foe.

5. It would be far better to refrain from killing such noble-minded teachers and to live in this world by begging for our food. Our teachers are desirous of wealth, but if we kill them the rewards we would then enjoy would be tainted with blood.

6. Nor do we know which would be better for us, defeating them or being defeated by them, for after killing the sons of Dhritarashtra who are now positioned before us, we would have no wish to live.

7. My very existence is afflicted by problems caused by weakness and my mind is confused about dharma. So now I am asking you which is the best course to adopt. Answer me clearly for I am now your student. Instruct me for I am surrendering to your guidance.

8. I cannot see anything that will dispel the grief that is drying

up my senses, not even attaining a prosperous kingdom on earth without any rival, nor even gaining lordship over the gods.

9. Samjaya said: After speaking in this way to Hrishikesha, Gudakesha said to Govinda, "I will not fight." He then fell silent, O destroyer of the foe.

10. With a slight smile, Hrishikesha then spoke these words to the lamenting Arjuna in the space between the two armies.

11. The Lord said: Grieving for that which should not be lamented over, you speak words that appear wise. But learned men grieve for neither the living nor the dead.

12. There was never a time when I did not exist, nor you, nor these lords of men; nor shall any of us cease to exist in the future.

13. For the embodied soul present in this body there is childhood, youth and then old age and in the same way it then acquires a different body. One who is wise is not confused about this.

14. It is contact with the senses, Kaunteya, which leads to sensations of heat and cold and pleasure and pain. Being impermanent, these sensations appear and then disappear and you must learn to endure them, Bharata.

15. If these sensations do not distract a person, O best of men, and he can remain equal in sorrow and happiness, then such a wise person gains the state of immortality.

16. That which is unreal never comes into being and that which is real never ceases to be. Those who perceive the truth can recognize this conclusion concerning these two.

APPENDIX

17. You must understand the indestructible principle that pervades this whole world. No one can bring about the destruction of this unchanging principle.

18. This embodied soul is eternal, indestructible and unlimited. The bodies it inhabits, however, must come to an end. Therefore fight, O Bharata.

19. Neither the person who thinks that this is the killer nor one who thinks it is killed properly understands it, for it does not kill and it cannot be killed.

20. It is never born and it never dies. It is existing now and it will never cease to exist. It is unborn, eternal, everlasting and most ancient. It is not killed when the body is killed.

21. How can a person who properly understands it as indestructible and eternal cause the death of anyone or kill anyone. What will he cause the death of? What will he kill?

22. Just as a man casts aside old clothes and puts on other ones that are new, so the embodied soul casts aside old bodies and accepts other new ones.

23. Weapons cannot cut it, fire cannot burn it, water cannot make it wet and wind cannot dry it.

24. This cannot be cut, it cannot be burned, and it cannot be moistened or dried. It is eternal, all-pervasive, fixed, immovable and everlasting.

25. It is said that it is imperceptible and inconceivable and it is not subject to transformation. Understanding it in this way, you should lament no more.

26. And even if you think that it is born repeatedly and repeatedly dies, still you should not lament over it, O mighty one.

I am confident, I can do it. Yes!!

27. For one who has been born death is certain and for one who has died, birth is certain. Therefore you should not lament over something that cannot be avoided.

28. In the beginning living beings are not manifest. They become manifest in the interim stage, Bharata, but at their end they become non-manifest again. Why should there be lamentation over this?

29. By some wonder a person may see it, by some wonder another person may speak of it and by some wonder yet another person may come to hear about it. But another person may not understand it even after hearing about it.

30. It is impossible to kill this embodied soul that is always present within the bodies of all beings. Therefore you should not lament over any living being.

31. Considering the nature of your own personal dharma, you should not hesitate. For a kshatriya there is nothing superior to fighting for the sake of dharma.

32. Kshatriyas who encounter a war of this type become joyful, Partha; it comes unsought and yet opens the door to heaven.

33. And if you do not engage in this dharmic battle then both your personal dharma and your honor will be destroyed and you will accumulate sin.

34. People will then speak of your everlasting dishonor and for a person who has achieved renown, dishonor is worse than death.

35. The great chariot warriors will think that you have left the battle due to fear. Those who had previously thought highly of you will now hold you in contempt.

APPENDIX

36. Your enemies will speak many insulting words about you, condemning your prowess. What could be more painful than that?

37. Either you will die and reach heaven or else you will conquer and rule the earth. Therefore arise, Kaunteya, with your resolve set on battle.

38. Become equal-minded towards happiness and distress, gain and loss, victory and defeat and then engage yourself in battle. You will never acquire sin by acting in this way.

39. I have spoken so far on the basis of Samkhya but now listen to this concerning Buddhi Yoga, the Yoga of the intellect. When you engage in action on the basis of this understanding (buddhya) you will free yourself from the bondage of action.

40. There is nothing to lose in this attempt and neither can there be any failure, for even a slight engagement in this dharma frees one from great danger.

41. Here the resolute intelligence becomes fixed on one point, O child of the Kurus, but the understandings of those who are irresolute have many branches and diversify without limit.

42. Persons lacking in insight who are attached to the religion of the Vedas speak in flowery language. "There is nothing more than this," they say.

43. Filled with desires and seeking the heavenly worlds they advocate many different types of rituals, which lead to a higher birth as the result of the action. Pleasure and power are the goals they seek.

44. The resolute form of intelligence existing in the state of samadhi can never arise for such persons who remain attached

to pleasure and power and whose minds are carried away by such desires.

45. The Vedas are permeated by the three gunas but you must become free of the three gunas, Arjuna. One who is self-possessed transcends duality, always adheres to the quality of Sattva and has no interest in gain or protection of property.

46. All the purposes served by a small reservoir of water can be fulfilled by a lake. In the same way the purposes served by all the Vedas are fulfilled for a Brahmin who is enlightened by knowledge.

47. You have a right to perform prescribed action but you are not entitled to the fruits of that action. Do not make the rewards of action your motive and do not develop any attachment for avoiding action.

48. Situated in Yoga, perform your actions, giving up all attachments, Dhanamjaya. Remain equal in success and failure for such equanimity is what is meant by Yoga.

49. Action (karma) is greatly inferior to Buddhi Yoga, Dhanamjaya. Seek shelter in the intellect (buddhau); those motivated by the fruits of action are petty-minded.

50. By engaging the intellect (buddhi-yukto) one sets aside both righteous and unrighteous deeds. Therefore engage yourself in this Yoga, for Yoga is the true art of performing action.

51. Wise men who engage in the Yoga of the intellect abandon the fruits that are born of action. Free from the bondage of which they attain a position that has no blemish.

52. When your intellect breaks free of the dense thicket of illusion you will reach a state of indifference for what should be

heard and what has been heard in the past (shruta).

53. Your intellect becomes perplexed by the Shruti, but when it remains steady and fixed in concentration without any wavering, you will then have achieved success in Yoga.

54. Arjuna said: What is the defining feature of a person whose realization is steady and who remains firm in his concentration, Keshava? How does such a steady-minded person speak? How does he sit? How does he move?

55. The Lord said: When a person sets aside all the desires running through his mind, Partha, and satisfies himself in the self alone he is then described as one whose wisdom is steady.

56. When the mind does not grieve over life's sorrows, when a person remains untouched by the joys of life and free of passion, fear and anger he is described as a sage whose understanding is steady.

57. When a person has no affection for any object at all and feels neither joy nor loathing when he gains desirable and unwanted results, then his wisdom is firmly established.

58. When a person withdraws all his senses from their objects, like a tortoise withdrawing its limbs, then his wisdom is firmly established.

59. The objects of pleasure do not touch the embodied soul who abstains from them. In this way one restricts one's inclination although the inclination remains, but after perceiving, the Supreme one completely renounces such desires.

60. The agitating senses can forcibly carry away the mind of even a perceptive person who makes the proper endeavors, Kaunteya

61. Restraining all these senses, one engaged in this practice should remain dedicated to me. When he has his senses under control then his wisdom is firmly established.

62. When a person thinks about the objects of the senses, attachment for them inevitably arises. Due to that attachment desire appears and from desire anger comes into being.

63. From anger comes delusion and as a result of that delusion one's memory is lost. When memory is lost one's intelligence is destroyed and when intelligence is destroyed a person is lost.

64. But one who possesses self-control can move amongst the sense objects using senses that are free of desire and loathing and are directed by his will alone. Such a person attains a state of absolute tranquility.

65. In that state of tranquility all his sufferings disappear. And when one's mind is thus at peace the realization then becomes steady.

66. But there can be no realization for one who does not engage in this practice and indeed no higher knowledge. Without that higher knowledge there is no peace and how can there be happiness without peace?

67. Whichever of the roaming senses the mind becomes attached to will carry away a person's understanding, just as the wind carries away a boat on the ocean.

68. Therefore, O mighty one, only if a person completely draws back his senses from their objects is his wisdom firmly established.

69. One who practices this restraint is awake when it is night

for all living beings. And that period in which living beings are awake is night for the perceptive sage.

70. Just as rivers flow into the sea, which is never filled and remains steady and immovable, so all these desires flow into such a person. It is he who attains peace, not one who seeks to fulfil those desires.

71. Giving up all desires such a person moves through life without attachment. He has no sense of 'mine' or 'I'; it is he who attains peace.

72. This is the transcendental state, Partha, and on reaching such a position one is no longer deluded. If one can remain situated in this state of consciousness even at the time of death then one attains Brahma Nirvana.

Chapter 3 (43 verses)

1. Arjuna said: If you regard realization as being superior to action then why are you urging me to engage in a form of karma that is so dreadful?

2. It seems that you are confusing my understanding by this equivocal instruction. Please tell me conclusively of the one course by which I can obtain the greatest benefit.

3. The Lord said: I have already explained, O sinless one, that in this world the path one should follow is twofold. For Samkhyas it is by the Yoga of knowledge and for Yogins it is by the Yoga of action.

4. A person does not gain freedom from action simply by ceasing to act and he cannot reach the ultimate state of perfection

by renunciation alone.

5. No one can remain still without performing any action, not even for a moment. Everyone is helplessly engaged in some form of action by the gunas that are born out prakriti (matter).

6. One who restricts his organs of action but continually dwells on the objects of the senses within his mind is a deluded soul. Such a person is referred to as a hypocrite.

7. But one who continues to act while controlling the senses within the mind, Arjuna, using his organs of action to perform Karma Yoga without any attachment, is certainly superior.

8. You should continue to perform your prescribed duties, for performing action is superior to refraining from action. You cannot even sustain your bodily functions without acting.

9. Except where action is performed in the execution of yajña, this world remains in the bondage of action. Remaining free of attachment, Kaunteya, you should therefore perform action for that purpose alone.

10. In the beginning, after creating living beings along with yajña, Prajapati said to them, "You will flourish by means of this ritual; this will be the cow that grants all your desires.

11. The gods are sustained in this way and those gods will then sustain all of you. Sustaining each other in this way, you will all achieve the highest benefit.

12. Sustained by yajña, the gods will bestow upon you all the food you may desire. One who consumes the foods given by the gods without making offerings to them is certainly a thief."

13. Righteous people who consume food left after a yajña are freed from all blemishes. But wicked people who cook just for

themselves eat food that is impure.

14. Living beings exist on food and food is produced due to rain. The rain comes as a result of yajña and yajña is performed by ritual action.

15. You should understand that ritual action is derived from the Veda (Brahma) and the Veda appears from the akshara (undecaying). Hence the all-pervasive Brahman is always present within the yajña.

16. In this world, a malicious person who delights only in the senses and does not perpetuate the cycle thus established certainly lives a worthless life.

17. But for a person who seeks pleasure in the self, finds contentment through the self and is fulfilled by the self there is no prescribed duty to perform.

18. There is nothing for him to gain by either performing or renouncing such duty. Nor is there any reason for him to be dependent on another living being.

19. Remaining always unattached, you should therefore perform your prescribed duty, for a person who performs such duty without attachment attains the highest goal.

20. It was through the performance of action that Janaka and others remained situated in a state of complete perfection. Just by considering the welfare of the world you should be inspired to act.

21. Whatever course of action a superior man pursues, lesser persons will follow and the world will accept the standard he sets.

22. There is no action that I am bound to perform anywhere in the three worlds, nor anything I might need that I have not

already attained, and yet still I am engaged in action.

23. For if ever I was to cease from the actions I so diligently perform, all people would follow my path, Partha.

24. If I did not perform these duties then these worlds would fall into ruin. I would then be the creator of children of mixed varnas and thereby cause harm to living beings.

25. People devoid of knowledge perform actions on the basis of worldly attachment, Bharata, and the wise should act in the same way, but without attachment—just for the welfare of the world.

26. The wise man should not cause any breach in the understanding of ignorant people who act on the basis of attachment. By acting while engaging in his Yoga discipline he should encourage them to perform all their duties.

27. All actions are ultimately performed by the gunas inherent in prakriti (matter), but a person whose mind is deluded by the sense of 'I' thinks, 'I am the doer.'

28. But one who understands the truth about the distinction between guna and action understands that it is just one set of gunas acting on other gunas. By understanding action in this way he remains unattached.

29. Those who are confused about the gunas inherent in prakriti have attachment for the action generated by the gunas. But one who understands all this should not disturb such ignorant persons who know nothing about it.

30. Casting off all your deeds onto me by fixing your mind on an understanding of the self and remaining free of desire and free of any sense of 'mine,' you should now fight with your

fever banished.

31. Persons who are faithful and devoid of envy and always adhere to the view I have just expounded are released from the effects of action.

32. But those who despise this teaching of mine and do not adhere to it are deluded in all their wisdom. You should know that they are lost souls who are completely dull-witted.

33. Even one who possesses knowledge conducts himself in accordance with his nature. Living beings must conform to nature so what will repression of one's nature achieve?

34. Desire and aversion are the conditions of the senses in relation to the objects they perceive. A person must not fall under the control of either of these tendencies, for both are obstacles to him.

35. Even though it may have faults, one's own dharma is still superior to accepting the dharma of another, even if it is perfectly observed. Death in the pursuit of one's own dharma is better, for another's dharma is a source of danger.

36. Arjuna said: What is it that impels a person so that he acts sinfully even though he has no desire to do so, Varshneya, compelling him to act in that way as if by force?

37. The Lord said: It is desire, it is anger; this arises from the guna known as Rajas. You should know this as a mighty devouring force, a great source of sin; it is the enemy in this world.

38. As fire is covered by smoke, as a mirror is covered by dirt and as an embryo is covered by its membrane, so is this world covered by desire.

39. Knowledge is covered by this desire, which is therefore the

great enemy of one who possesses knowledge. This enemy has the form desire, Kaunteya, and blazes like an insatiable fire.

40. The senses, the mind and the intellect are said to be its abode. Covering the true knowledge of the embodied being, it then places it in a state of delusion.

41. Therefore you must first regulate the senses, O best of the Bharatas, and then conquer this source of sin, which destroys both spiritual and practical knowledge.

42. They say that the senses are in a superior position and that the mind is superior to the senses. The intellect stands above the mind, but this is superior even to the intellect.

43. Thus understanding that which is superior to the intellect and making yourself steady by your own means, you must defeat this enemy in the form of desire, O mighty one, for it is difficult to overcome.

Chapter 4 (42 verses)

1. The Lord said: I instructed this unfading Yoga to Vivasvan. Vivasvan instructed it to Manu and Manu taught it to Ikshvaku.

2. The Raja-Rishis (royal saints) thus understood this Yoga, receiving it one from the other in succession. After a long time had passed in this world, knowledge of this Yoga was lost, Paramtapa.

3. This same ancient Yoga has today been instructed by me to you. You are my devotee (bhakta) and my friend. Therefore this most profound mystery (is revealed to you).

4. Arjuna said: Your birth was later than the birth of Vivasvan,

APPENDIX

which was earlier. So how can I accept that you taught this to him in the beginning?

5. The Lord said: There are many births of mine that have passed and of yours also, Arjuna. I know about them all but you do not know of them, Paramtapa.

6. Although I am unborn and my identity is unchanging, although I am the controller (ishvara) of all beings, still I resort to my prakriti energy and I appear by means of my own power.

7. Whenever there is a decline in dharma, O Bharata, and whenever there is an increase in adharma, then I manifest myself.

8. For the protection of the righteous (sadhus), for the destruction of the wrongdoers and for the purpose of establishing dharma, I appear age after age.

9. One who fully understands this truth about my divine birth and activity does not take birth again after giving up his body. He goes to Me, Arjuna.

10. Free of desire, fear and anger, wholly dedicated to me and dependent upon me, many persons purified by knowledge and austerity have attained my state of existence.

11. To the degree that they become dependent upon me so I devote myself to them. In all circumstances people follow the path I set for them, Partha.

12. Seeking success through ritual action they worship the gods. In the human sphere, it is quickly attained through ritual acts.

13. I created the system of four varnas, based on the gunas and types of action. And although I am the creator of this system,

you should understand that I am still the one who does not act, the one who does not decay.

14. Actions cannot leave a mark on me and I am unaffected by the fruits of action. One who understands this truth about me is not bound by the actions he performs.

15. In the past this truth was well known to people who sought liberation from rebirth and hence they performed action. So you should also perform your designated actions, just as people in the past fulfilled their duties.

16. What is action? What is inaction? Even learned scholars are confused about this. I will now explain to you what action is; when you understand this you will be freed from everything that is impure.

17. One must understand about action and one must understand about forbidden action. One must also understand what inaction is; the course of action is indeed hard to comprehend.

18. One who perceives inaction in action and action in inaction is intelligent among men. He is properly engaged and he performs all his designated actions.

19. When all a person's endeavors are devoid of any inclination toward desire, his action is burned by the fire of knowledge. The wise ones describe such a person as a learned pandit.

20. When a person gives up attachment for the fruits of action, he is always satisfied and is not dependent on any other; he performs no action at all even though he is engaged in action.

21. By remaining free of expectations, controlling his thoughts, practicing self-control, giving up all desire for acquisitions and acting only for the maintenance of the body, a person remains

free of contamination.

22. If he is satisfied with whatever befalls him, transcends duality, is free of envy and is equal in success and failure, then even though he engages in action he is not bound by it.

23. For a liberated person whose attachments have vanished, whose mind is absorbed in higher knowledge and who acts only in the form of yajña, any action he performs dissolves away completely.

24. The sacrificial offering is Brahman. The oblation is Brahman; it is offered by Brahman into the fire that is also Brahman. Brahman alone is reached by a person who absorbs his mind completely in the ritual act that is Brahman.

25. Some practitioners make yajña offerings dedicated to the gods alone but others make their offerings into the fire of Brahman, performing yajña for its own sake.

26. Then there are some who offer hearing and the other senses into the fires of restraint and others who offer sound and the other objects of the senses into the fires of the senses themselves.

27. Others offer the actions performed by the senses and the movements of the breath into the fire of Yoga practice based on self-control, which is lit by means of true knowledge.

28. Some sages, strictly adhering to their vows, perform yajña through certain objects, some through religious austerity, some through Yoga and some through recitation and knowledge of sacred texts.

29. Others offer the prana breath into the apana and the apana into the prana, dedicating themselves to the practice of

pranayama by restricting the movement of the prana and the apana.

30. Others restrict their eating and make offerings of the prana breaths into the prana breaths themselves. All such persons who have knowledge of yajña have their contaminations destroyed by means of yajña.

31. Consuming the nectar or immortality in the form of the leftover offerings at the end of a yajña, they proceed to the eternal region of Brahman. There is nothing in this world for a person who performs no yajña, O best of the Kurus, but this is even truer of the other world.

32. Thus many different types of yajña are expanded within the mouth of Brahman. You must understand that all of them are based on action, for when you understand this you will be liberated.

33. The Jñana Yajña, consisting of knowledge, is superior to the Dravya Yajña, consisting of physical objects, O destroyer of the foe. Without any exception, Partha, all action finds its proper conclusion in knowledge.

34. You should gain this knowledge through submission, inquiry and service. Those who have knowledge and perceive the truth will then impart knowledge to you.

35. And when you have acquired this knowledge, you never again fall prey to illusion, Pandava, for you will see that all living beings are within your own self and moreover within me.

36. Even if you perform sinful acts more heinous than those of all other sinners, still you can cross beyond all such wickedness by means of the boat of knowledge.

37. Just as a blazing fire turns fuel to ashes, Arjuna, so the fire of knowledge turns all actions to ashes.

38. In this world there is nothing as purifying as knowledge. In due time, a person who is successful in Yoga practice will find this knowledge within himself through himself alone.

39. One who has faith will acquire this knowledge if he devotes himself to the quest and gains mastery over the senses. And when he has acquired this knowledge he very soon attains supreme peace.

40. A doubting soul, devoid of faith and knowledge, meets with destruction. Neither this world nor the world to come is for the doubting soul and he can never be happy.

41. When his action is given up to the practice of Yoga, when his doubts are destroyed by knowledge and when he is in full control of his existence, a person's actions cannot bind him, Dhanamjaya.

42. Therefore, using the sword of knowledge, cut through this uncertainty of yours that has arisen due to ignorance and is now situated in your heart. Take up this Yoga and arise, Bharata.

Chapter 5 (29 verses)

1. Arjuna said: Krishna, you advocate both the renunciation of action and the yoga of action as well. But which of these is the better course? Tell me this definitively.

2. The Lord said: Renunciation and Karma Yoga both lead to the highest result. But between the two, Karma Yoga is superior to

the renunciation of action.

3. One who neither loathes nor hankers after anything is to be known as a constant renunciant. Remaining free of duality, O mighty one, he easily breaks free of bondage.

4. Foolish children say that Samkhya and Yoga are different, but not learned pandits. A person who properly adheres to one of these paths gains the fruit of both.

5. The position achieved by the followers of Samkhya is also attained by those who adhere to the path of Yoga. One who sees that Samkhya and Yoga are one and the same truly sees.

6. But without engaging in Yoga practices, renunciation is very difficult to achieve. The sage who engages in Yoga practice quickly attains Brahman.

7. One who engages in Yoga and has purified his very being, who has gained self-mastery and control of the senses, whose own self has become the self of all beings, is not besmirched even though he engages in action.

8. One who is engaged in Yoga practice and sees the truth thinks, "I never perform any action." He thinks in this way even while seeing, hearing, touching, eating, moving, sleeping, breathing,

9. Speaking, evacuating, seizing, opening his eyes or closing them, he considers, "It is just the senses engaging with their objects."

10. One who deposits his actions on Brahman and abandons attachment is not smeared by sin when he acts, as a lotus leaf is not touched by water.

11. Abandoning attachment, yogins then act with body,

mind and speech, or just with the senses, in order to purify themselves.

12. Abandoning the fruits of action, the practitioner of Yoga attains enduring peace. But one who does not engage in Yoga and is motivated by desire remains in bondage, attached to the fruits of action.

13. Giving up all actions within the mind, the embodied being remains joyful and in full control within the city of nine gates, neither acting nor causing action to be performed.

14. The Lord generates neither the means by which action is performed nor the actions themselves as performed by the people of the world. Nor does he create the conjunction between action and its result; it is a person's inherent nature that does this.

15. The mighty Lord does not assume anyone's sin or indeed their virtue. But knowledge is covered over by ignorance and so living beings become deluded.

16. But for some people, the ignorance shrouding the inner self is destroyed by knowledge. For such persons, knowledge acts like the sun and illuminates the higher reality.

17. Their intelligence, their life and their conviction are devoted to that goal, for they are fully dedicated to it. Purged of contamination by means of knowledge, they go to the place from which there is no return.

18. The learned pandit regards with equal vision a Brahmin endowed with wisdom and good conduct, a cow, an elephant, a dog and one who eats dogs.

19. Even while they are still in this world, persons whose minds

are fixed in this state of equanimity conquer the process of creation. Brahman is free of blemish and always the same, and so they are situated in Brahman.

20. Such persons do not rejoice when they gain what is dear to them nor are they disturbed when they experience something undesirable. Their intellect is steady, they are free of delusion, they have knowledge of Brahman and they are situated in Brahman.

21. Remaining unattached to external sensations, such a person finds joy in the self within. Absorbing himself in Brahman through Yoga practice, he experiences joy that does not decay.

22. The pleasures that arise from sensual contacts are in fact sources of misery. They have a beginning and an end, Kaunteya, and so an enlightened person (budha) does not delight in them.

23. Any person in this world who is able to resist the force of desire and anger before being released from the body is indeed a Yogin and a joyful man.

24. One whose happiness is within, whose pleasure is within and whose light is within is indeed a Yogin. Being situated in Brahman, he attains the state of Brahma Nirvana.

25. Rishis who are free of contamination gain that state of Brahma Nirvana. Their sense of duality is destroyed, they are self-controlled and they take delight in the welfare of all beings.

26. This Brahma Nirvana quickly arises for sages detached from desire and anger whose minds are controlled and who have knowledge of the inner self.

27. Setting aside external perceptions and fixing his vision between the eyebrows, bringing the prana and apana breaths into a state of equilibrium as they move within the nostrils,

28. And controlling the senses, mind and intellect. The sage who constantly dedicates himself to liberation from rebirth, giving up desire, fear and anger, is indeed a liberated person.

29. Understanding me to be the enjoyer of yajña and acts of austerity, the supreme lord of all the worlds and the friend of all beings, he attains a state of absolute tranquility.

Chapter 6 (47 verses)

1. A person who performs the action he is duty-bound to perform, remaining detached from the fruit of action, is a true renunciant and a Yogin, not one who never lights the sacrificial fire and does not perform the ritual.

2. You should know that that which they call renunciation is in fact Yoga, Pandava. One who has not given up the inclination for pleasure can never become a Yogin.

3. For the sage who is a beginner in Yoga, action is said to be the means, but for one who is advanced in Yoga tranquility is said to be the means.

4. When he has no attachment for the objects of the senses or for performing action and he gives up all material inclinations, he is said to be advanced in Yoga.

5. One should elevate oneself by oneself alone and one should never degrade oneself. One is indeed one's only friend and one's own enemy as well.

6. The self is the friend to one who is self-controlled by means of personal commitment. But when one has lost his self, then the self acts with hostility like an enemy.

7. For a person who has self-control and possesses inner tranquility, the supreme self is realized, whether it be in heat or cold, happiness or distress, honor or dishonor.

8. Satisfied by his knowledge and realization alone, situated in a higher position, mastering his senses, one who engages in this way is said to be a Yogin. He regards lumps of earth, stones and gold equally.

9. When considering friends, allies, enemies, those who are indifferent, neutrals, those who hate one, relatives, righteous persons and the wicked, an equal mind is superior.

10. The Yogin should engage himself constantly, staying in a secluded place. He should remain alone, controlling his mind and himself, without any aspiration and without any sense of ownership.

11. He should prepare a firm seat for himself in a pure place, not too high and not too low, covered with cloth, animal hide and kusha grass.

12. Sitting there on his seat, fixing his mind on a single point, controlling the movements of his thoughts and senses, he should engage in Yoga practice in order to purify himself.

13. Holding his body, head and neck in a straight line, steady and without moving, he should concentrate on the point of his nose while not looking in any direction.

14. With his whole being in a state of tranquility, free of fear, accepting the vow of celibacy, controlling his mind, with his

APPENDIX

thoughts concentrated on me, the practitioner should sit there, dedicating himself to me.

15. Constantly engaging himself in this way, the Yogin who controls his mind attains tranquility, the ultimate Nirvana, which is my state of being.

16. Yoga cannot be practiced if one eats excessively or does not eat at all, nor if one sleeps too much or remains constantly awake.

17. The Yoga that destroys suffering can be practiced if one properly engages one's eating, leisure pursuits, performance of action, sleeping and wakefulness.

18. When a person fixes the controlled mind on the atman alone, untouched by any desires, he is then said to be properly engaged.

19. Yogins who have controlled their minds and practice Yoga in relation to the atman have been compared to a lamp in a windless place that never flickers.

20. When the restrained mind ceases from its activities due to the practice of Yoga and when the atman is perceived by means of one's own faculties, then a person finds satisfaction within the atman.

21. When one experiences that limitless joy, which is grasped by the intellect but is beyond the range of the senses, one remains fixed on it and never wavers from that truth.

22. After attaining this state one realizes that there is no level of achievement superior to it. When situated in this state of being, one cannot be disturbed even by terrible suffering.

23. One should understand that what is known as Yoga

amounts to the breaking of the connection with suffering. Yoga must be performed with firm resolve and with a state of mind free of despondency.

24. This should be done while giving up all the desires that arise from one's material inclinations and restraining the entire group of senses by means of the mind alone.

25. One should undertake this withdrawal little by little, using the resolutely focused intellect. Fixing the mind in conjunction with the atman, one should not think of any other object.

26. One must withdraw the wavering, unsteady mind from wherever it wanders and bring it back under control, fixed on the atman alone.

27. The highest joy comes to that yogin whose mind is tranquil, whose passions are quieted, who exists as Brahman and who has no blemish.

28. Engaging himself constantly in this pursuit, the yogin who is free of blemish easily makes contact with Brahman and acquires endless joy.

29. One who engages in Yoga practice sees the atman within all beings and all beings within the atman, maintaining this equal vision everywhere.

30. For one who sees me everywhere and who sees everything as existing within me, I am never lost, nor is he ever lost to me.

31. Regardless of the way he lives, one who adheres to this sense of oneness and worships me as being situated within all beings is a yogin who exists in me.

32. One who sees everything in relation to the self, Arjuna,

and thus regards pleasure and suffering as the same, is considered to be the highest yogin.

33. Arjuna said: I see no firm status for the Yoga you have explained in relation to equal-mindedness, Madhusudana, because of this unsteadiness.

34. The mind is unsteady, Krishna, it is dominating, powerful and harsh. I think controlling the mind is harder to achieve than controlling the wind!

35. The Lord said: Without doubt, O mighty one, the mind is flickering and difficult to restrain. But it can be restrained through constant endeavor and renunciation, Kaunteya.

36. In my opinion, it is difficult for a person who lacks self-control to follow the path of Yoga. But one who makes this endeavor after achieving self-mastery is able to do so by employing the proper means.

37. Arjuna said: A person who does not endeavor enough but is endowed with faith may be distracted from Yoga by the fluctuations of the mind and so fail to gain the goal of Yoga. What result does he achieve, Krishna?

38. With both his aims unachieved, is he not lost like a divided cloud without any real position, O mighty one, deluded from the path to Brahman?

39. You should completely dispel this doubt of mine, Krishna. Except for yourself there is no one who is able to dispel it.

40. The Lord said: Neither here nor in the next world, Partha, is such a person ever lost. No one who does good ever attains a bad result thereby.

41. After reaching the worlds enjoyed by the righteous and

residing there for innumerable years, the failed yogin takes birth in the house of pure-hearted, fortunate people.

42. Or he may be born into a family of yogins, possessed of wisdom. In this world a birth of that type is very rarely attained.

43. In that family he regains the state of consciousness he achieved in his previous body and once more endeavors for perfection, O child of the Kurus.

44. He is helplessly drawn in that direction due to the regulated practice he previously undertook. Even a person who merely attempts to gain an understanding of Yoga transcends the teachings of the Veda.

45. Due to his endeavor, the yogin, engaged in his practice and purified of faults, gains perfection after several births and then goes on to the highest destination.

46. The yogin is superior to one who undertakes austerity. He is also regarded as being superior to one who possesses knowledge and to one performs ritual action. Therefore, Arjuna, become a yogin.

47. And of all yogins, he who has faith and who worships me with his inner self absorbed in me is engaged in the best practice. That is my opinion.

Chapter 7 (30 verses)

1. The Lord said: Now hear, O Partha, how you can have full knowledge of me without any doubts by fixing your mind upon me and practicing Yoga dedicated to me.

2. I shall explain to you in full both the Iñana and the vijñana.

APPENDIX

When this is understood there is nothing else remaining that should be known.

3. Among thousands of men only one will endeavor for perfection, and among those who do endeavor for perfection only one will come to know me in truth.

4. Earth, water, fire, air, space, mind, intellect and the sense of ego, comprise the eight components of my energy known as prakriti.

5. This is the inferior prakriti, but you should also know about my higher prakriti, which is distinct from it. This is the jiva bhuta, O mighty one, by means of which this world is held in place.

6. You should understand that these two are the origin (womb) of all living beings. I am the source of the entire world and its passing away as well.

7. There is no other thing that is superior to me, Dhanamjaya. This whole world rests on me just as jewels rest on their thread.

8. I am flavor in water, Kaunteya. I am the effulgence of the moon and the sun. I am Pranava (Om) in all the Vedas, I am sound in space and manliness in men.

9. And I am the primal aroma in earth; I am the heat in fire. I am life in all living beings; I am the religious austerity of those who undertake such austerities.

10. You should know me as the eternal seed of all beings, Partha. I am the intelligence of those who are intelligent; I am the energy of all energetic sources.

11. And I am the power of the powerful when it is devoid of desire and passion. I am desire in living beings, O best of the

Bharatas, when it does not transgress dharma.

12. You should understand that the states of existence based on Sattva, Rajas and on Tamas come into being from me. But I am not in them; they are in Me.

13. Being deluded by these three states of being, which are based on the three gunas, the whole world cannot understand me, for I am beyond all three states and I am undecaying (avyaya).

14. This divine maya of mine, consisting of the gunas, is difficult to go beyond. Only those who surrender to me cross beyond this maya.

15. The wrongdoers, the foolish, the lowest of men, persons whose knowledge is taken away by illusion (maya) and those who take to the asuric form of existence do not surrender to Me.

16. Four types of righteous persons worship Me, Arjuna: one who is in distress, one who wishes to understand, one who seeks prosperity and the jñanin who possesses knowledge, O best of the Bharatas.

17. The one possessing knowledge (jñanin) who is always properly engaged and has one-pointed devotion is the best of these. I am very dear to such a jñanin and he is dear to me.

18. They are all noble persons, but I regard the jñanin as my very self (atma). He is situated so as to dedicate himself to me as his ultimate goal.

19. At the end of many births, one who possesses knowledge surrenders to me, realizing, "Vaasudeva is all things." Such a mahatma is very rarely found.

20. Pursuing this or that desire, those who lack knowledge

APPENDIX

surrender to other gods, accepting the appropriate discipline for worship as dictated by their own inner nature.

21. Whatever the divine form that the devotee wishes to faithfully worship, I bestow upon him the firm faith that enables him to do so.

22. When he is endowed with that faith, he then engages in the worship of that god and as a result attains what he desires. These desired objects are, however, granted by me.

23. But the results of the worship performed by such unintelligent persons are all temporary. The worshippers of the gods go to the gods; my devotees go to me.

24. Those who lack intelligence think of me as being a non-manifest entity taking a manifest form. They do not know my higher nature, which is unfading and unsurpassed.

25. Being covered by yogamaya, I am not manifest to all. So this deluded world does not comprehend me, the one who is unborn and unfading.

26. I know the living beings of the past, the present and the future, Arjuna, but there is no one who knows me.

27. Through the illusion of duality, Bharata, arising from desire and loathing, all living beings pass into a state of ignorance in this created world, Paramtapa.

28. But persons whose wickedness has reached an end and who are engaged in virtuous acts become free from the illusion of duality. They worship me and remain firm in their vows.

29. Those who resort to me and thereby endeavor for liberation (moksha) from old age and death fully understand Brahman, and have complete knowledge of adhyatma and of

action (karma).

30. Those who also know me in relation to the adhibhuta, the adhidaiva and the adhiyajña can, with their consciousness fixed, know me even at the time of death.

Chapter 8 (28 verses)

1. Arjuna said: What is that, Brahman? What is adhyatma? What is karma, O Purushottama? And what is it that is referred to as adhibhuta? What is it that is called adhidaiva?

2. What is adhiyajña, O Madhusudana, and how is it present within this body? And how are you to be known at the time of death by those who have attained self-mastery?

3. The Lord said: That which decays not (akshara) is the Supreme Brahman; it is one's inherent nature (sva-bhava) that is referred to as adhyatma. The creative force producing the existence of living beings is known as karma.

4. Adhibhuta is the existence that decays, and adhidaiva is the soul within (purusha). I alone am the adhiyajña here in this body, O best of embodied beings.

5. And one who leaves the body at the time of death while remembering me attains my existence. There is no doubt about that.

6. Whatever the state of being a person's mind is fixed upon at the time of death as he leaves his body is the state he then attains, Kaunteya, for a person develops into the type of existence he constantly exists as.

7. At all times therefore you should think of me and engage

APPENDIX

in battle. If your mind and intellect are fixed on me, you will undoubtedly come to me.

8. It is through the consciousness being absorbed without deviation in the disciplined practice of Yoga that a person goes to the Supreme Divine Being upon whom his thoughts are fixed.

9. One should absorb the mind in him, thinking of him as the ancient seer, the controller who is smaller than the smallest thing, the ordainer of all that comes to pass, whose form is inconceivable, who is like the sun in color and who is beyond all darkness.

10. At the time of death a person should absorb himself in devotion (bhakti) with an unwavering mind, using the power of Yoga practice. Placing the life air between the eyebrows in the proper way, he thus attains that original Supreme Person.

11. I shall now fully explain to you that position which those who know the Vedas speak of as the akshara (undecaying) and which sages who are devoid of passion enter into. It is due to their desire for this position that they take vows of celibacy.

12. It is by sealing all the entrances of the body, by holding the mind steady on the heart and keeping the air of life at the top of the head that a person becomes fixed in Yoga concentration.

13. A person who gives up his body and departs this world while reciting 'Om,' which is the one imperishable (akshara) Brahman, and remembering me attains the highest destination.

14. For a person who always sets his mind on me and never allows his concentration to wander, who is a yogin constant in his practice, I am very easy to attain, Partha.

I am confident, I can do it. Yes!!

15. Rebirth is miserable and temporary, but after attaining me, the mahatmas never take birth again, having achieved the highest state of perfection.

16. Repeated birth occurs in all the worlds from Brahmaloka downwards, Arjuna. But after attaining Me, Kaunteya, there is no more rebirth.

17. Those persons who understand his day and his night recognize the limit of Brahma's day as one thousand yugas (ages) and they understand his night as also lasting for a thousand yugas.

18. When the day commences, all beings emerge from their non-manifest state and become manifest. When the night comes, they merge once more into that which is known as the non-manifest.

19. Coming into being time and again, this host of living beings is helplessly merged back once more when the night comes. And at the coming of the day they appear again.

20. Beyond that state of non-manifestation, however, there is another non-manifest state of existence, which is eternal. When all living beings are destroyed, that state is not destroyed.

21. They describe this supreme destination as non-manifest and non-decaying (akshara). On reaching this position one does not return. It is my supreme abode.

22. That Supreme Being, Partha, is attained by undivided devotion. The living beings are situated within him and he pervades the whole world.

23. Now, O best of the Bharatas, I shall speak of the time of

departing in which the yogins do not return to this world and the time in which they do return.

24. Persons who have knowledge of Brahman (or the Vedas) and depart during the fire, the light, the day, the moon's light fortnight, or the six months when the sun is in the north go to Brahman.

25. But a yogin who departs during the smoke, the night, the dark fortnight of the moon or the six months when the sun is in the south come back to this world after entering the light of the moon.

26. Thus it is believed there are two paths from this world, the light and the dark. By following one there is no return, but by following the other one he comes back once more.

27. Understanding these two paths, Partha, the yogin is never bewildered. So engage yourself in Yoga practice at all times, Arjuna.

28. A specific reward is ordained as the fruit of the merit (punya) acquired through study of the Vedas, sacrifice (yajña), religious austerity (tapa) or acts of charity, but the yogin goes beyond all of that. Completely understanding the wisdom I have revealed, the yogin goes to the original, supreme position.

Chapter 9 (34 verses)

1. But now, O non-envious one, I will reveal to you this greatest of mysteries, which includes both jñana and vijñana. When this is understood you will be liberated from unwanted things.

2. This teaching is the king of knowledge, the king of mysteries. This is the purest of all things. It can be understood by direct perception, it is based on dharma, it is very easy to perform and it is unfading.

3. Persons who have no faith in this dharma do not attain Me, Paramtapa. They return to the path of death and rebirth.

4. This whole world is pervaded by me in my non-manifest form. All beings are situated in me but I am not present in them.

5. And yet the living beings are not situated in me; you should see this as my magical opulence. My identity is what causes living beings to exist; it sustains the living beings but is not situated within them.

6. The great wind that always moves through all places is situated in space. You should understand that it is in this sense that all living beings are situated in me.

7. At the end of the period of creation (kalpa), Kaunteya, all beings enter into My prakriti energy and at the beginning of a kalpa, I manifest them again.

8. Making use of my own prakriti energy, I repeatedly create this entire host of living beings. They are powerless for they are under the control of prakriti.

9. And these actions do not bind me, Dhanamjaya. I am situated in a position of apparent neutrality, unattached to these actions.

10. It is through me alone that prakriti brings the moving and non-moving beings into existence, for I am the Controller. This is the designated cause by means of which the world proceeds

on its course.

11. Fools despise me when I accept this human form. They do not understand my higher identity as the Supreme Lord of the living beings.

12. The hopes, deeds and understanding of these unintelligent persons are futile. Falling prey to delusion they adopt the nature of asuras and rakshasas.

13. But the mahatmas resort to the divine nature, Partha. Having understood that I am the origin of all beings, they worship me with undeviating minds.

14. Constantly singing my praises, engaging in resolute vows and bowing before me with devotion, they are always engaged in acts of worship.

15. Others make offerings through the jñana-yajña, the sacrifice of knowledge, and worship me as He who is one and yet many and whose manifold faces turn in every direction.

16. I am the ritual, I am the sacrifice, I am the oblation offered to the ancestors and I am the herbs. I am the mantras, I alone am the ghee, I am the sacred fire and I am the offering made into the fire.

17. I am the father of this world, the mother, the ordainer and the grandfather. I am the object of knowledge, I am that which is pure, I am the syllable om, and I am the Rig, the Sama and the Yajus.

18. I am the goal, the sustainer, the lord, the witness, the abode, the refuge and the friend. I am creation, destruction and maintenance, I am the treasury and I am the unfading seed.

19. I bring forth warmth, I hold back the rain and I then release it. I am immortality and I am death. I am both being and non-being, Arjuna.

20. Drinking Soma, purged of sin (papa), those who follow the three Vedas seek the heavenly destination after worshipping me with yajñas. Acquiring piety (punya) in this way they attain the world of the lord of the gods and in that heaven they enjoy the celestial pleasures enjoyed by the gods.

21. But after enjoying the delights of that wonderful heavenly domain, they must re-enter the mortal world when their stock of piety (punya) becomes exhausted. So by adhering to the dharma of the three Vedas, persons who seek to fulfil their desires gain only a temporary reward.

22. Then there are persons who worship me with undeviating concentration. For those who engage constantly in this way I bring both prosperity and security.

23. Those who are devoted to other gods and worship them with faith actually worship me alone, Kaunteya, but not in the manner that is properly ordained.

24. I am the enjoyer and also the master of all yajñas. Such persons do not know me as such and so fall down from the position they attain.

25. Devotees of the gods go to the gods, devotees of the ancestors go to the ancestors, those who worship spirits go to the spirits but those who worship me go to me.

26. When it is presented in a mood of devotion I will accept the devotional offering of a leaf, a flower, a fruit or water from one who possesses self-mastery.

APPENDIX

27. Make whatever you do, whatever you eat, whatever you sacrifice, whatever charity you give, and whatever austerities you undertake into an offering to Me, Kaunteya.

28. In this way you will be liberated from the auspicious and inauspicious results, the bonds of action. Engaged in this Yoga of renunciation, you will become liberated and you will come to me.

29. I am equal toward all living beings; no one is hated by me and no one is beloved. Those who worship me with devotion, however, are in me and I am in them.

30. Even if a person who worships me as his only object is a performer of the most wicked deeds, still he is to be considered a sadhu, for his resolution is correct.

31. He quickly becomes a dharmatma, committed to dharma, and attains enduring peace. Make it known, Kaunteya, that my devotee does not perish.

32. Having sought shelter with me, Partha, even those of evil birth as well as women, vaisyas and shudras go to the highest destination.

33. How much more so then in the case of the Brahmins, the righteous (punyah), the devotees and the religious kings (raja-rishis). So having reached this temporary world that is devoid of happiness, you should engage in worshipping me.

34. Fix your mind on me, become my devotee, worship me and bow down to me. By engaging yourself in such acts and dedicating yourself to me, you will surely come to me.

I am confident, I can do it. Yes!!

Chapter 10 (42 verses)

1. The Lord said: Listen again, O mighty one, to the excellent words I will speak to you. You have love for me and I desire your welfare.

2. The gods cannot comprehend my origin and neither do the great rishis. Indeed it is I who am the source of all the gods and all the great rishis.

3. One who knows me as unborn and without beginning, the great Lord of the worlds, is the one who is not deluded among mortal beings. He is liberated from all sins.

4. Intelligence, knowledge, freedom from illusion, tolerance, truthfulness, self-control, tranquility, joy, misery, existence, non-existence, fear, fearlessness,

5. Not harming, equanimity, satisfaction, austerity, charity, fame and infamy are states of existence for living entities and these varied categories of being arise from me alone.

6. In the beginning the seven great rishis and the four Manus come into being from me by means of my thoughts, and the living beings existing in the world are all produced by my thoughts as well.

7. One who properly understands this glory and mystical power of mine engages in unwavering Yoga discipline. There is no doubt about this.

8. I am the origin of all things; everything comes into being from out of me. When they understand this, the enlightened ones worship me, filled with loving attachment.

9. Their minds are absorbed in me, their lives are given over to me, and they enlighten one another about me. Talking

APPENDIX

constantly about me, they find satisfaction and delight.

10. To those who engage constantly in this way, worshipping in a mood of love, I give that yoga of the intellect by means of which they come to me.

11. I am situated in their own existence and, due to my compassion, I destroy the darkness that arises from ignorance with the blazing torch of knowledge.

12. Arjuna said: You are the Supreme Brahman, the supreme abode and the most pure. You are the eternal divine purusha, the original Deity, unborn and almighty.

13. All the rishis speak of you in this way, including Narada the divine rishi, Asita, Devala and Vyasa. Now you yourself are declaring it to me.

14. I accept everything you have said to me as true, O Keshava. Neither the gods nor the Danavas (asuras) can understand your manifestation, O Lord.

15. You alone can understand your own Self by your own power, O Supreme Person, for it is through you that living beings exist. You are the Lord of all beings, the god of gods, the Lord of the world.

16. You should now fully explain your own divine glories. Tell me about those glorious attributes through which you pervade these worlds and remain present within them.

17. How are you to be thought of, O yogin, when I constantly fix my mind upon you? In what forms of existence can I think of you, O Lord?

18. Speak to me again, Janardana, about your extensive Yoga and glorious power (vibhuti). When hearing this nectar I am

never fully satiated.

19. The Lord said: Very well, I will speak about my own divine attributes, but only those that are most prominent, O best of the Kurus, for there is no end to my extent.

20. I am the atman, Gudakesha, situated in the hearts of all beings. I am the beginning of the living beings and I am their middle and end as well.

21. Among the Adityas I am Vishnu, among luminous objects I am the radiant sun. Among the Maruts I am Marichi and among stars I am the moon.

22. Of the Vedas I am the Sama Veda, among the gods I am Vasava (Indra). Among the senses I am the mind and among living beings I am consciousness.

23. Among the Rudras I am Shankara, among the Yakshas and Rakshasas I am Vittesha. Among the Vasus I am fire (Agni) and among mountain peaks I am Meru.

24. Priests know me to be Brihaspati, the foremost of them. Among generals I am Skanda and among lakes I am the ocean.

25. Among the great rishis I am Bhrigu, among sounds I am the one syllable (om). Among yajñas I am the Japa Yajña and of things that move not, I am Himalaya.

26. Among all the trees I am the Ashvattha (fig) tree, among the divine rishis I am Narada. Among the Gandharvas I am Chitraratha and among those who have achieved perfection I am Kapila Muni.

27. Among horses, know me to be Ucchaihshravasa who appeared from the nectar. Among the lords of the elephants I am Airavata and among men I am the king.

APPENDIX

28. Among weapons I am the thunderbolt, among cows I am the kamadhuk. Among progenitors I am Kandarpa and among serpents I am Vasuki.

29. Among the Nagas I am Ananta, among those who inhabit the waters I am Varuna. Among the ancestors I am Aryama and among those who subdue others I am Yama.

30. Among the Daityas I am Prahlada, among those who calculate I am time. Among beasts I am the king of the beasts and among birds I am Vainateya (Garuda).

31. Of purifiers I am the wind, among those who bear weapons I am Rama. Among the fish I am the Makara and among rivers I am Jahnavi (Ganga).

32. Among creations I am the beginning and end and I am the middle as well, Arjuna. Of all forms of knowledge I am knowledge of the atman and among debaters I am the ultimate conclusion.

33. Among letters I am the letter "a", among compound words I am the dual word. I am time that has no end and I am the Ordainer whose faces turn in all directions.

34. I am death who carries everyone away, I am the origin of all things yet to be. Among women I am fame, good fortune, speech, memory, intelligence, endurance and forgiveness.

35. Of the Sama hymns I am the Brihat Sama, of the hymns of the Veda I am the Gayatri. Of the months I am Margashirsha and of the seasons I am that which brings the flowers.

36. Among cheats I am dicing, I am the energy of those who possess energy. I am victory, I am resolution and I am the existence of all that exists.

37. Among the Vrishnis I am Vaasudeva (Krishna), among the Pandavas I am Dhanamjaya (Arjuna). Amongst sages I am Vyasa and among seers I am the seer named Ushanas.

38. Among those who chastise I am punishment, among those who seek victory I am good policy. Among secrets I am silence and I am the knowledge of those who possess knowledge.

39. And I am that which is the seed of all living beings, Arjuna. There is no living being, moving or non-moving, which exists except through me.

40. There is no end to my divine glories and attributes, O Paramtapa, but I have revealed this much just as an indication of the extent of my glory.

41. You should understand that whenever a glorious form of existence displays its opulence or power, it arises from a small part of my energy.

42. But what is the need for you to understand it to such an extent, Arjuna? Just know that I am present here, sustaining the whole world with just a part of myself.

Chapter 11 (55 verses)

1. Arjuna said: For my benefit you have explained the ultimate mystery, which is known as the adhyatma. Through this explanation my illusion is now gone.

2. I have heard from you at length about the beginning and end of the living beings, O lotus-eyed one, and about your unfading power.

3. You are certainly what you have described yourself to be, O

Parameshvara, and I now wish to behold that glorious form of yours, O Purushottama.

4. If you think it is possible for me to see it, O Lord, then reveal to me your unfading Self, O Yogeshvara.

5. The Lord said: Behold, O Partha, my hundreds and thousands of divine forms; they are of various different types, of many colors and forms.

6. Behold the Adityas, Vasus, Rudras, Ashvins and Maruts, numerous things that have never before been seen. Behold these wonders, O Bharata.

7. Today behold the entire world with its moving and non-moving creatures here in one place, O Gudakesha, and whatever else you wish to see.

8. But you are not able to see this with your own eyes, and so I give to you divine vision. Now behold my glorious Yoga!

9. Samjaya said: When he had spoken these words, O king, Hari the great lord of Yoga revealed to Partha His supreme, glorious form.

10. It had many mouths and eyes and many features wonderful to behold. It had many divine ornaments and many divine weapons raised aloft.

11. It was adorned with celestial garlands and garments and was anointed with celestial perfumes. This limitless Deity was entirely wondrous and his faces turned in all directions.

12. If a thousand suns were to rise in the sky, each with a blazing effulgence, it might then resemble the brilliant radiance of that great being.

13. The Pandava then saw the entire world, undivided and yet manifold, situated there in one place within the body of the god of gods.

14. Thereupon Dhanamjaya became filled with wonder and the hairs on his body stood erect. Bowing his head to that Deity and placing his palms together, he then said,

15. Arjuna said: I see all the gods in your body, O Lord, and the entire host of living beings. I see Brahma, the lord, who remains seated on a lotus, and all the rishis and celestial serpents.

16. With so many arms, bellies, mouths and eyes, I see you with this unlimited form that is everywhere. There is no end, no middle and no beginning as I behold you, for you are the Lord of the world and the world is your body (vishva rupa).

17. I see you with a crown, club and disc and your fiery effulgence illuminates all directions. I see you everywhere though you are so difficult to look upon for the blazing light of fire and sun spreads beyond measure.

18. You are to be known as the Supreme Akshara (undeteriorating). You are the ultimate abode of this world. You are unfading (avyaya), the eternal guardian of dharma and I regard You as the eternal purusha.

19. You are without beginning, middle or end and have limitless power. You have unlimited arms and the sun and moon are your eyes. I see you with blazing fire coming from your mouth as you heat this entire world with your own energy.

20. The heavens, the earth and the sky are pervaded by you alone and so are all the directions. After seeing this wonderful

and yet terrible form of yours, the three worlds are trembling, O Mahatma.

21. These hosts of celestial beings are entering into you; some are afraid and praise you with folded palms. The hosts of rishis and perfect beings proclaim the sound svasti, (let it be good) and glorify You with hymns and words of praise.

22. The Rudras, Adityas, Vasus, Sadhyas, Vishva-devas, Ashvins, Maruts, ancestors, Gandharvas, Yakshas, Asuras and Siddhas are all beholding you in astonishment.

23. This great form of yours has many mouths and eyes, O mighty one, and has many arms, thighs and feet. It has many bellies and many fearsome teeth. After seeing this form the worlds tremble in fear and so do I!

24. Your multicolored effulgence reaches the limit of the sky, your gaping mouths are wide open and your wonderful eyes are blazing. Seeing you thus, my inner self is trembling with fear; I cannot maintain my steadiness or composure, O Vishnu.

25. Seeing your faces with their terrible teeth, which are like the fire at the end of the world, I can no longer recognize the directions or understand my position. Become my refuge and show your grace, O Lord of the gods who is the abode of the world.

26. All these sons of Dhritarashtra along with this host of kings, as well as Bhishma, Drona, the suta's son and the great warriors of our army as well

27. Are all rushing forth and entering your mouths with those terrible teeth that are a cause of fear. Some of them can be seen caught between those teeth with their heads being crushed.

I am confident, I can do it. Yes!!

28. As the many currents of the rivers rush with force and flow toward the ocean, so these heroes among men enter your blazing mouths.

29. As insects meet with destruction by rapidly entering a burning lamp, so the worlds rush forward and meet with destruction by entering your mouths.

30. Devouring the worlds from all sides, you lick them all up with your blazing mouths. Having filled the entire universe with its energy, this terrible effulgence of yours is scorching everything, O Vishnu.

31. Tell me who you are with this fearful form. I bow down to you, be merciful, O greatest of the gods. I wish to know your original identity. I cannot comprehend this activity of yours.

32. The Lord said: I am the time that matures and brings destruction to the world. My activity is to draw in the worlds. Except for yourselves none of these warriors drawn up in ranks will survive.

33. Therefore arise and win renown. Having defeated your enemies you may enjoy a prosperous kingdom. These warriors are already slain by me and you should be my instrument, Savyasachin.

34. Drona, Bhishma, Jayadratha, Karna and the other heroic warriors have been killed by me. You will conquer so do not waver. Wage war and you will defeat your enemies in the battle.

35. Samjaya said: After hearing Keshava's words, Kiritin joined his palms and paid his respects while trembling in fear. He then addressed Krishna again in stuttering tones, paying his

respects in a mood of awe and fear.

36. Arjuna said: As is appropriate, Hrishikesha, the world is delighted by your glorification and becomes joyful. While the terrified rakshasas will flee in various directions, the hosts of perfect beings will bow down before you.

37. Why should they not bow before you, O Mahatma, for you are greater even than Brahma, the original creator of the world? You are the unlimited lord of the gods, the abode of the world; you are the aksharam, (that which does not deteriorate) and you are that which lies beyond both being and non-being.

38. You are the original Deity, the primeval purusha. You are the final resting place of this world. You are the knower and the known, the supreme, the abode. This entire world is pervaded by You, O You of limitless form.

39. You are Vayu, Yama, Agni, Varuna, the Moon, Prajapati and the grandfather. I bow to you, I bow to you a thousand times over and then still I bow to you once again.

40. I bow to you from the front, I bow from behind and I bow from all sides, for you are everything. Your power is unlimited and your might cannot be measured. It is you alone who can achieve all things and therefore you are all things.

41. Thinking of you as a friend, I spoke presumptuously, saying, "O Krishna, O Yadava, O my friend, I was unaware of your greatness and I did this out of folly or perhaps out of affection.

42. Making jokes, I behaved improperly toward you while we were passing time together, resting, sitting or eating, sometimes when we were alone and sometimes in the sight of

others, Achyuta. Now I beg your forgiveness for you are beyond all measure.

43. You are the father of the moving and non-moving world; you are the object of worship for the world and you are the greatest teacher. No one is your equal and no one is greater than you in all the three worlds, for your power is unrivalled.

44. Therefore I bow down to you and prostrate my body. I seek your grace for you are the worshipful Lord. Please tolerate my conduct, O Lord, as a father to a son, a friend to a friend, or a lover to his beloved.

45. I am pleased to have seen this form that was never previously seen but my mind has been disturbed by fear. Now show me that other form, O Lord. Show me mercy, O lord of the gods, abode of the world.

46. I now wish to see you with a helmet, a club and a disc in your hand. O thousand-armed one, O Vishva Murti, please now assume that four-armed form.

47. The Lord said: It is with pleasure, Arjuna, that this supreme form has been displayed by me by means of my own Yoga. It is filled with energy, it is the world, it is unlimited and original. It has never been displayed by me to anyone but yourself.

48. Not through the Veda, yajña, recitation, charity, ritual or harsh austerity can I be seen in this form in the world of men by anyone other than you, O hero of the Kurus.

49. Do not tremble with fear and do not be bewildered after seeing this form of mine, which is so fearful. Let your fears be dispelled and let your mind be contented once more; now behold that form of mine.

APPENDIX

50. Samjaya said: After speaking to Arjuna in this way, Vasudeva again displayed his own form. The Mahatma stilled Arjuna's fear by again assuming his benign form.

51. Arjuna said: Seeing this benign human form of yours, Janardana, my mind is now at peace and I have regained my normal condition.

52. The Lord said: This form of mine that you have seen is very hard to gain a vision of. Even the gods are always longing for a vision of this form.

53. Not through the Vedas, austerity, charity or sacrifice is it possible to see me in the way that you have seen me here.

54. But through devotion to me alone, Arjuna, it is possible to know me and to see me in this form and indeed to enter into me, Paramtapa.

55. One who performs his deeds for me, dedicates himself to me as my devotee, remains free of attachments and has no hatred for any living being, will come to Me, Pandava.

Chapter 12 (20 verses)

1. Arjuna said: Between those devotees who dedicate themselves to you, being constantly engaged in the way you have described, and those who revere the non-manifest akshara feature, who are superior in Yoga?

2. The Lord said: In my opinion, those who fix their minds on me, who constantly engage in serving me and who possess absolute faith are engaged in the best way possible.

3. But those who dedicate themselves to the non-deteriorating

(akshara), indeterminate, non-manifest feature, which is present everywhere, is unknowable, and is situated in the transcendent realm, unmoving and constant,

4. Who regulate all their senses and who have the same attitude toward everyone also attain me, delighting as they do in the welfare of all beings.

5. But there is greater difficulty involved for those whose thoughts adhere to the non-manifest feature. The way to the non-manifest feature is one of suffering for embodied beings.

6. But for those who are devoted to me, who dedicate all their actions to me, who meditate on me and worship me through single-pointed Yoga,

7. I become without delay the Uplifter from the ocean of death and rebirth, for their consciousness is absorbed in me.

8. Set your mind on me alone; let your intellect enter into me. You will then dwell in me alone, of this there is no doubt.

9. If you are not able to hold your consciousness steadily upon me, then you should seek to attain me by means of regulated Yoga practice, O Dhanamjaya.

10. If you are unable even to perform this regulated practice, then dedicate yourself to working on my behalf. By performing acts on my behalf, you will still achieve the goal.

11. And if you are unable to undertake the practice of Yoga dedicated to me, then gain self-control and perform the renunciation of the fruits of all action.

12. Knowledge is better than regulated practice and meditation is superior to knowledge. Renouncing the fruits of action is better than meditation and unending tranquility is superior

APPENDIX

to renunciation.

13. Having no hatred for any living being, goodwill, compassion; having no sense of possession, no pride, remaining equal in misery and joy, and being merciful;

14. Being always satisfied, being a yogin who possesses self-control, who is firm in his commitment and who has absorbed his mind and intelligence in me: such a devotee is loved by me.

15. From whom the world has no fear and who does not fear anyone in the world, who is free from elation, distress, fear and passion; such a person is loved by me.

16. Who has no hankerings, is pure, expert, indifferent, free of anxiety and who has renounced his material endeavors; such a devotee is loved by me.

17. Who does not rejoice or hate, lament or hanker, and who has renounced both pleasing and vile objects; such a devoted one is loved by me.

18. Who is equally disposed toward an enemy and a friend, who regards respect and contempt as the same, who is the same in heat or cold and in joy and misery and who has given up all attachment to the world,

19. Who is unmoved by condemnation or praise, who is silent and satisfied with whatever comes his way, who has no permanent abode, and is steady in his understanding; such a devoted one is loved by me.

20. Those who venerate the nectar of the dharma I have spoken of here and who have full faith and are dedicated to me are my devotees and they are certainly loved by me.

Chapter 13 (34 verses)

1. The Lord said: This body, Kaunteya, is referred to as the kshetra (field) and those who possess this wisdom know that which has knowledge of the field as the kshetrajña, the knower of the field.

2. You should also understand that I am the kshetrajña present within all the kshetras, Bharata. In my opinion, knowledge of the kshetra and kshetrajña is knowledge indeed.

3. So listen to me now as I explain briefly about the kshetra and what it is like, about the transformations it undergoes and about which one of them comes from the other. I will also explain who he is and what his powers are.

4. This subject has been sung about by the rishis in many ways in the various hymns of the Veda. It has also been explained with reasoned conclusions in the aphorisms of the Brahma Sutra.

5. The great elements, the sense of ego (ahamkara), the intellect, matter in its non-manifest state, the eleven senses and the five objects they perceive,

6. Desire, loathing, joy, misery, the aggregate of all faculties, consciousness and resolve; this is what is known as the kshetra, outlined in brief, along with the transformations it undergoes.

7. Avoiding pride and deceit, not harming, patience, honesty, serving the acharya, purity, steadfastness, self-control,

8. Detachment from the objects of the senses, being free of the sense of ego, perceiving the problem inherent in the misery of birth, death, old age and disease,

9. Being unattached and without affection for sons, wife and

home, always maintaining an equal disposition whatever happens, be it desirable or undesirable,

10. Maintaining undeviating devotion to me through Yoga that is fixed on no other point, living in a deserted place, taking no pleasure in other people's company,

11. Constant dedication to the knowledge designated as adhyatma, perceiving the true object of knowledge; this is said to be jñana (knowledge) and everything else is said to be ajñana (ignorance).

12. I shall now speak about the jñeya, the object we must strive to know, for when this is known one attains immortality. It is without beginning, it is the Supreme Brahman (or it is without beginning and dependent on me); it is said that it is neither existent nor non-existent.

13. Its hands and feet are everywhere, its eyes, heads and mouths are everywhere, its ears are everywhere in the world; thus it remains pervading all things.

14. It appears to have the attributes of senses and yet in truth it is devoid of senses. It is without attachment but it supports all things, it is free of the gunas and yet it experiences the gunas.

15. It is both outside and within the moving and non-moving beings. Because of its subtle nature it is hard to know, it is far away but very close as well.

16. It appears to be divided up within different living beings and yet it remains undivided. That jñeya, which must be known, sustains living beings, it devours them and it brings them into being as well.

17. It is the light of luminous objects and is said to be beyond

the darkness. It is knowledge, the object that should be known, and it is accessible through knowledge; it is situated within the heart of all beings.

18. Now kshetra, jñana and jñeya have all been briefly explained. After realizing this truth, my devotee attains my state of existence.

19. You should understand that both prakriti and purusha have no beginning. You should also know that all transformations and the gunas have their origin in prakriti.

20. In terms of the enactment of the process of cause and effect, prakriti is said to be the ultimate cause while in the experiencing of joy and misery, purusha is said to be the cause.

21. While situated within the domain of prakriti, the purusha experiences the attributes that are born of prakriti. Attachment to these attributes is the cause of the purusha's birth in both auspicious and inauspicious wombs.

22. He is the witness and the one who grants permission, the sustainer, the enjoyer, the great Lord (maheshvara). He is referred to as paramatman (the higher self) and within the body he is the supreme purusha.

23. One who thus understands purusha and prakriti, along with its gunas, never takes birth again even though he is active in many different ways.

24. By means of the self, some perceive the self within themselves through meditation. Others do this through the Yoga of Samkhya and others again through Karma Yoga.

25. Then there are still others who do not gain knowledge by any of these means but devote themselves to the self after

hearing from other people. Dedicating themselves to learning in this way, they too cross beyond death.

26. Every form of existence, moving or non-moving, that comes into being should be understood as arising from a combination of kshetra and kshetrajña, Bharata.

27. The supreme Lord is equally present in all living beings. When the body is destroyed he is not destroyed. One who perceives this existence truly sees.

28. A person who perceives the same Lord situated everywhere will not harm the self by means of the self. As a result of this realization he goes to the supreme abode.

29. All types of action are performed by prakriti alone. One who thus sees that the atman is not the performer of action truly sees.

30. When a person sees the manifold existence of living beings situated as one entity and that they expand from out of that one entity, he then attains Brahman.

31. Because it is without beginning and is untouched by the gunas, even though it is situated within the body this unchanging paramatman does not act and is not contaminated.

32. Just as the all-pervasive space is never contaminated due to its subtle nature, so the atman situated everywhere within the body is not contaminated.

33. And just as the sun alone illuminates this whole world, so the dweller in the field illuminates the entire kshetra, Bharata.

34. Persons who possess the eye of knowledge can comprehend the distinction between kshetra and kshetrajña and the liberation of living beings from prakriti. Such persons reach the supreme.

Chapter 14 (27 verses)

1. Once more I will speak to you about the highest knowledge, which is supreme among all types of knowledge. All those sages who comprehend this wisdom depart from here and achieve the highest perfection.

2. Devoting themselves to this knowledge, they come to my own state of being. Hence they are not born at the time of creation and at the time of destruction they are not disturbed.

3. My womb is the great Brahman and I deposit an embryo therein. The origin of all beings arises from out of this union, Bharata.

4. Different forms appear in all the various wombs, Kaunteya, but the great Brahman is the womb for them all and I am the father who bestows the seed.

5. Sattva, Rajas and Tamas are the gunas arising from prakriti. They bind the changeless, embodied entity that exists within the body, O mighty one.

6. Due to its being free from blemish, wherever Sattva exists there is illumination and no contamination. It is through attachment to happiness and attachment to knowledge (jñana) that it causes bondage, O sinless one.

7. You should understand that Rajas is of the nature of passion; it becomes prominent due to hankering and attachment. It binds the embodied entity through attachment to action, Kaunteya.

8. And you should know that Tamas, which is delusion for all embodied beings, appears due to ignorance. It causes bondage through negligence, idleness and sleep.

9. Sattva causes one to adhere to happiness while Rajas causes

APPENDIX

adherence to action, Bharata, and by obscuring a person's wisdom Tamas creates adherence to negligence.

10. Sattva prevails by subjugating Rajas and Tamas, Bharata; Rajas prevails by subjugating Sattva and Tamas, and Tamas prevails by subjugating Sattva and Rajas.

11. When the illumination of knowledge appears in all the doorways in this body, you should realize that Sattva has become dominant.

12. Greed, endeavor, engagement in activities, agitation, hankering; these appear when Rajas becomes dominant, O best of the Bharatas.

13. Dullness, inaction, misunderstanding, delusion; these appear when Tamas becomes dominant, O child of the Kurus.

14. When the embodied soul encounters death while Sattva predominates, it then moves on to the pure worlds obtained by those who possess higher knowledge.

15. If he meets with death while Rajas predominates, he takes birth among those attached to action and if he dies while Tamas predominates he is reborn within the wombs of those whom he deluded.

16. They say that the fruits of righteous deeds are Sattvic and without blemish. But suffering is the fruit of Rajas and ignorance is the fruit of Tamas.

17. Knowledge arises from Sattva and greed arises from Rajas. Negligence, delusion and ignorance arise from Tamas.

18. Those who adhere to Sattva move upwards, those who adhere to Rajas remain in between, while those who adhere to Tamas and follow the ways of the lowest guna go downward.

I am confident, I can do it. Yes!!

19. When the observer sees that there is no actor other than the gunas and gains knowledge of that which is beyond the gunas, he attains my state of being.

20. Transcending these three gunas that cause the body to exist, the embodied entity is liberated from the misery of birth, death and old age and attains immortality.

21. Arjuna said: What are the characteristics of one who has transcended these three gunas, O Lord? How does he behave? How does he go beyond the three gunas?

22. The Lord said: He does not hate illumination, activity or delusion when they appear, Pandava, and neither does he long for them when they disappear.

23. He is one who remains indifferent and is not disturbed by the gunas, who thinks, "It is the gunas alone that are active." He thus remains steady and does not waver.

24. He is equally disposed in distress and happiness, he is self-contained, and he views a lump of earth, a stone and gold as the same. He is firmly resolved and he is equally disposed toward dear ones and strangers, toward criticism and glorification.

25. Whether honored or condemned he is still the same, and he is equally disposed toward friends and foes. He has abandoned all his worldly endeavors. Such a person is said to be beyond the gunas.

26. And one who reveres me through undeviating Bhakti Yoga also transcends the gunas and becomes fit to attain the Brahman existence.

27. For I am the foundation on which the immortal, unchanging

Brahman exists. I am also the foundation of the eternal dharma and of absolute joy.

Chapter 15 (20 verses)

1. The Lord said: They speak of an unfading Ashvattha tree with its roots above, its branches below and the Vedic hymns as its leaves. One who understands this tree has knowledge of the Vedas.

2. Its branches spread out above and below, nourished by the gunas. The objects of the senses are its shoots. Its roots also spread down below where they become combined with action in the human domain.

3. Its form cannot be identified for it has no end and no beginning and no foundation either. Using the strong weapon of detachment, one should cut down this Ashvattha tree with its fast sprouting roots.

4. One should then seek that position from which, once it is attained, there is no return, thinking, "I surrender to that original being (purusha) out of whom the primeval creative impulse flowed forth."

5. Without pride or folly, conquering the problem of attachment, constantly absorbed in knowledge of the atman, with desires restrained, free from the duality identified as pleasure and suffering, those who are free of illusion then progress to that changeless state of being.

6. The sun does not illuminate that place, neither does the moon or fire. Having gone there one does not return; that is

my supreme abode.

7. In the world of living beings (jiva-loka), the eternal living element is nothing but a part of me. It draws to itself the five senses and the mind, which is the sixth, all of which rest on prakriti.

8. When the Lord (ishvara) takes on a body and then moves on from it, he holds on to these six in the way the wind carries aromas from their original place.

9. Making use of the senses of hearing, sight, touch, taste and smell, as well as the mind, he then experiences the objects of the senses.

10. Whether he is departing or remaining, or whether he is experiencing the world by association with the gunas, those who are deluded do not perceive him. Those, however, who possess the eye of knowledge can perceive him.

11. Yogins who pursue their endeavors perceive him situated within their own being, but those who are unintelligent and fail to achieve self-mastery will never perceive him despite making the endeavor.

12. The energy centred in the sun, which illuminates the entire universe, and that of the moon and fire as well—that energy is mine alone.

13. Entering into the earth, I sustain the living beings through my potency. Becoming the moon, which is imbued with liquid potency, I nourish all the plants.

14. I become the Vaishvanara energy, the digestive heat, and reside in this form within the bodies of the living beings. By combining with the prana and apana breaths, I digest the four types of food.

APPENDIX

15. And I am situated in the hearts all; memory, knowledge and the loss of knowledge arise from me. It is I who am to be understood from all the Vedas. I am the creator of Vedanta and it is I who understands the Vedas.

16. In the world there are these two purushas, the kshara (decaying) and the akshara (non-decaying). The kshara is all living beings, while that which is in a higher position is referred to as akshara.

17. But the highest purusha is different again and is designated as the paramatman. This is the unfading Lord who enters the threefold world and sustains it.

18. And because I am beyond the kshara and superior to the akshara as well, I am therefore celebrated in both the world and in the Veda as 'Purushottama'.

19. One who is not deluded and knows me thus as purushottama, knows all things. He then worships me with his entire existence, O Bharata.

20. I have now proclaimed this most secret of teachings, O sinless one. One who comprehends this doctrine is wise indeed and has fulfilled his responsibilities, O Bharata.

Chapter 16 (24 verses)

1. Fearlessness, purification of one's nature, remaining resolute in the pursuit of knowledge through Yoga practice, charity, self-control, performing sacrifices, recitation of the Vedas, austerity, honesty;

2. Not harming, truthfulness, avoiding anger, renunciation,

tranquility, never maligning others, compassion for other beings, being free of greed, kindness, modesty, never wavering;

3. Energy, patience, resolve, purity, the absence of malice and of arrogance; these constitute the daivi sampad, the godly disposition, of one who is born with this nature, Bharata.

4. Deceit, arrogance, pride, anger, harshness and ignorance are the asuri sampad, the asuric disposition, of one who is born with that nature, Partha.

5. The daivi sampad leads to liberation but the asuri sampad is regarded as a cause of bondage. Do not be concerned, you have been born with the daivi sampad, Pandava.

6. There are two manifestations in this world, the daiva and the asura. I have described the daiva at some length so now hear from me about the asura disposition, Partha.

7. Asuric persons know nothing about the performance of ritual action or about the renunciation of action. Neither purity nor good conduct are ever found in them, nor indeed is truthfulness.

8. They say, "The world has no permanent truths, it has no absolute basis and no presiding Deity. It comes into being without any causal sequence. Where is there any causal factor apart from lust?"

9. Those who have destroyed their souls and have little intelligence adhere to views of this type. Inimical to all, they then engage in cruel deeds that bring destruction to the world.

10. Pursuing desires that are difficult to fulfil, filled with deceit, pride and passion, they adhere rigidly to their false conceptions and proceed on the basis of impure resolve.

All I want is within me now,

APPENDIX

11. Right up to the point of death they are beset by limitless anxieties, devoting themselves to the fulfilment of sensual desires, convinced there is nothing more.

12. Bound by hundreds of ropes in the form of their aspirations, dominated by desire and anger, they accumulate wealth by immoral means in order to fulfil their desires.

13. "I have obtained this much today and I will obtain more to satisfy my desire. This much wealth is mine now and this much will come to me in the future.

14. I have slain this enemy and I will kill the others as well. I am the Lord, I am the enjoyer, I am successful, powerful and happy.

15. I am wealthy and born into a good family. Who is there who can be my equal? I will perform sacrifices, I will give charity and thus I will rejoice." Such are the ideas of those deluded by ignorance.

16. Being distracted by so many different notions, entangled in the net of delusion, and addicted to the enjoyment of their desires, they fall down into an impure state of hell.

17. Being full of self-importance, stubborn, and dominated by wealth, pride and passion, they perform rituals that are yajña in name only, deviating from the prescribed method due to their deceitful nature.

18. Absorbing themselves in egotism, strength, arrogance, desire and anger, they display hatred and envy toward me, present as I am in their own bodies and in the bodies of others as well.

19. Those cruel persons are filled with hatred and are the

lowest of men. I perpetually cast such impure beings into asura wombs in the cycle of rebirth.

20. Entering an asuric womb birth after birth, such fools never attain me, Kaunteya, and so they move on to the lowest state of being.

21. This doorway to hell that destroys the soul is threefold, consisting of desire, anger and greed. You should therefore renounce these three.

22. A man who frees himself from these three gateways of Tamas, Kaunteya, can act for his own welfare and then proceed to the highest abode.

23. One who abandons the rules ordained by scripture and acts according to his own desire can never attain perfection, happiness or the highest abode.

24. Therefore scripture should be your authority in establishing what should and should not be done. And when you understand the rules revealed by scripture, you should act in accordance with your duty.

Chapter 17 (28 verses)

1. Arjuna said: There are some people who faithfully make spiritual endeavors but ignore scriptural rules. What is their position, Krishna? Is it said to be in Sattva, Rajas or Tamas?

2. The Lord said: The faith of embodied beings arises from their inherent nature and is of three types. It can be based on Sattva, Rajas or Tamas. Now hear about this.

3. For all beings, the faith they have corresponds to their

APPENDIX

nature, Bharata. A person is pervaded by his faith, for the nature of that faith shapes what he is.

4. Those who are Sattvic worship the gods, those dominated by Rajas worship yakshas, and rakshases and persons under the influence of Tamas worship spirits and ghosts.

5. Some people who undertake acts of austerity perform ferocious deeds not prescribed by scripture. They are motivated by hypocrisy and egotism and are beset by the power of desire and passion.

6. Such fools simply cause the elements of the body to waste away and they harm myself as well, for I am also present in the body. You should understand them as having the conviction of the asura nature.

7. Now the food that all beings find pleasing is also of three types, as is yajña, austerity and charity. Listen to this analysis of those categories.

8. The foods liked by Sattvic persons are those that bring long life, vigor, strength, health and which cause happiness and delight. Such foods are very tasty, juicy, crisp and pleasing.

9. Foods that are liked by persons predominated by Rajas are bitter, sour, salty, very hot, pungent, strong-tasting and burning. Such foods cause suffering, sorrow and ill-health.

10. The food liked by those predominated by Tamas is generally stale, tasteless, rotten, left over, dirty and foul.

11. When yajña is performed without desire for any result, in strict accordance with the proper rule, and with the mind absorbed in the thought, "It is a duty to make this offering," then it is of the nature of Sattva.

12. But when it is performed with some result in mind or out of hypocrisy, O best of the Bharatas, that yajña is of the nature of Rajas.

13. And when it is performed without regard for the proper rules, without food offerings, chanting of the hymns, payment to the priests, or any real faith in the process, they say that yajña is of the nature of Tamas.

14. Austerity of the body is said to consist of worship of the gods, Brahmins, teachers and wise men, cleanliness, honesty, celibacy and not harming (ahimsa).

15. Austerity of speech is said to consist of speaking words that do not disturb and that are true, loving and beneficial, as well as the regular recitation of the Vedas.

16. And austerity of the mind is said to consist of mental serenity, benevolence, silence, self-control and a pure disposition.

17. When men engaged in Yoga practice undertake this threefold austerity with the highest faith and without desire for any result, that austerity is said to be of the nature of Sattva.

18. But when the austerity is undertaken for the sake of respect, reputation and worship, or with hypocrisy, it is said to be of the nature of Rajas and is wavering and unsteady.

19. And that austerity by which one inflicts pain on oneself due to foolish notions or which is intended to bring destruction to others is declared to be of the nature of Tamas.

20. Charity that is given with the thought, "This should be given" and is presented to a suitable recipient from whom nothing is expected in return at the right time and place is of the nature of Sattva.

21. But that charity which is given with the expectation of getting something in return, for some subsequent result, or with reluctance is of the nature of Rajas.

22. And that charity which is given at the wrong place and wrong time to an unsuitable recipient, which is given improperly and with contempt, is of the nature of Tamas.

23. The words "Om Tat Sat" are understood as a threefold representation of Brahman. It was with this mantra that the Brahmins, Vedas and yajñas were established in ancient times.

24. Therefore the followers of the Veda always recite the syllable 'om' when they perform ritual acts of yajña, charity and austerity, in accordance with the prescribed rule.

25. Without desire for the fruit of their action, persons who seek liberation from rebirth recite the syllable 'tat' when they perform various ritual acts of yajña, austerity and charity.

26. This term 'sat' is used to designate both existence and righteousness. The word 'sat' is also used in the performance of sacred rituals, Partha.

27. In yajña, austerity and charity 'sat' is spoken of as meaning perseverance. And the ritual action by which these are performed is also designated as 'sat.'

28. If an act is performed without faith, be it a sacrificial offering, a gift in charity or act of austerity, it is then referred to as 'a-sat,' Partha. It has no effect either in the world to come or here in this world.

Chapter 18 (78 verses)

1. Arjuna said: I wish now to learn about the subject of samnyasa, O mighty one, and, Hrishikesha, about the distinction between samnyasa and tyaga, O slayer of Keshin.

2. The Lord said: Learned men understand samnyasa to be the giving up of action motivated by selfish desire. The wise further define tyaga as the renunciation of the fruits of action.

3. Some of those endowed with wisdom assert that action must be abandoned because it is inherently flawed. But others say that ritual acts of yajña, charity and austerity must not be abandoned.

4. Now hear my verdict on this debate over renunciation, O best of the Bharatas. Renunciation has been declared to be of three types, O tiger among men.

5. The ritual acts of yajña, charity and austerity must not be abandoned. Rather they should be performed, for it is yajña, charity and austerity that purify men of wisdom.

6. Renouncing attachment and the fruits of action, one must perform these ritual actions. This is my ultimate conclusion, Partha.

7. The renunciation of prescribed action is improper. The renunciation of such action due to delusion is proclaimed to be of the nature of Tamas.

8. If action is given up as painful, due to fear of the suffering it might cause to one's body, that renunciation is of the nature of Rajas and one will not gain the fruit of renunciation in that way.

9. But if one thinks, "This must be performed" and then completes his prescribed duty while renouncing attachment and

the fruits of action, Arjuna, that renunciation is known to be of the nature of Sattva.

10. The renouncer who is predominated by Sattva does not loathe action even when it is not pleasing and neither is he attached to pleasant action. He is a wise man whose doubts are dispelled.

11. It is impossible for anyone who has a body to completely give up action, but one who renounces the fruits of action is said to be a true renouncer.

12. Undesirable, desirable and mixed are the three types of result that come from action. After death these befall those who are not renounced but never those who are renounced.

13. Now learn from me about these five causal factors, O mighty one, established by the Samkhya system as determining the results of all actions.

14. These are the place of action, the performer, the various instruments employed and the different acts performed. Destiny is then the fifth factor.

15. Whatever action is undertaken with body, words or mind, be it proper or perverse, these five are its causes.

16. As this is the case, anyone who, due to his uneducated understanding, sees the self alone to be the performer of action has the wrong idea and does not see at all.

17. If a person has no sense of being the performer of action and if his consciousness is not absorbed in the action, then even if he destroys all these worlds he does not kill and he is not bound.

18. Knowledge, the object that is known and the one who knows, represent the threefold impulse for action. The

instrument, the deed and the performer represent the three constituents of an action.

19. Knowledge, action and the performer of action are all threefold according to the gunas. This can be shown by analysis in relation to the gunas so now listen to the way these are arranged.

20. When one changeless existence is seen in all beings, undivided in their diverse forms, you should know that knowledge to be of the nature of Sattva.

21. But when knowledge displays an understanding based on distinction and recognizes various types of existence of different forms, you should know that knowledge to be of the nature of Rajas.

22. And that knowledge which for no apparent reason attaches itself to a single cause as if it were everything, which is unaware of the truth and which is thus limited in scope is regarded as being of the nature of Tamas.

23. Action that is prescribed is performed without attachment and is undertaken without passionate endeavor, hatred or desire for the fruits is said to be of the nature of Sattva.

24. But action performed due to hankering for a desired object out of a sense of pride or with excessive endeavor is regarded as being of the nature of Rajas.

25. And action undertaken due to folly, and without regard for consequences, damage, violence or valor is said to be of the nature of Tamas.

26. When he is free of attachment, never speaks with any sense, is endowed with resolve and fortitude, and is unmoved by success or failure, the performer of action is said to be of

the nature of Sattva.

27. But if he is desirous and seeks the fruit of action, is greedy, violent by nature and impure, and is beset by feelings of delight and lamentation, that performer of action is regarded as being of the nature of Rajas.

28. And that performer of action who is negligent, vulgar, obstinate, deceitful, vicious, indolent, uninspired and procrastinating is said to be of the nature of Tamas.

29. Now hear about the threefold division of intelligence and of resolve in relation to the gunas, which I shall fully explain to show the differences between them, Dhanamjaya.

30. That which understands prescribed action, the renunciation of action, what should and should not be done, what is to be feared and what is not, as well as bondage and liberation is intelligence under the influence of Sattva.

31. But that by which dharma and adharma are not clearly understood, nor indeed prescribed duty and forbidden action, is intelligence under the influence of Rajas, Partha.

32. But that intelligence which is covered by ignorance and so thinks adharma to be dharma and has wrong conceptions on all subjects is intelligence under the influence of Tamas.

33. That resolve by means of which one sustains the activities of the mind, breath and senses in undeviating Yoga practice is of the nature of Sattva.

34. But that resolve by which a person who is attached to the world and seeks the results of action adheres to dharma, fulfilment of desire and the gaining of prosperity is of the nature of Rajas.

35. And that resolve due to which a fool does not break free from sleep, fear, grief, depression and intoxication is of the nature of Tamas.

36. Happiness is also of three types. Now hear from me, O best of the Bharatas, about how a person finds joy due to his repeated practice and thereby puts an end to sorrow.

37. That which is like poison in the beginning but at the end is like nectar is said to be happiness of the nature of Sattva. It arises due to the clarity of one's intellect.

38. But that happiness which is obtained through the contact of the senses with their objects and is like nectar in the beginning but like poison in the end is understood to be of the nature of Rajas.

39. And that happiness which is delusion for the self in both the beginning and the end, based on sleep, indolence and stupidity, is of the nature of Tamas.

40. Neither on earth nor in the heavens among the gods is there any form of existence that is free of these three gunas, which are born of prakriti.

41. The duties of Brahmins, kshatriyas, vaishyas and shudras, O scorcher of the foe, are designated in accordance with the gunas that arise from their inherent nature.

42. Tranquility, restraint, austerity, purity, patience, honesty, theoretical knowledge, practical knowledge and acceptance of the Vedic revelation are the actions of a Brahmin, born of his inherent nature.

43. Heroism, energy, resolve, expertise, never fleeing from battle, charity and displaying a lordly disposition are the

actions of a kshatriya, born of his inherent nature.

44. Agriculture, tending cows and trade are the actions of a vaishya, born of his inherent nature, while work consisting of service to others is the action of a shudra, born of his inherent nature.

45. A man can attain perfection by devoting himself to his own particular duty. Now hear how one who dedicates himself to his specific duty achieves that perfect state.

46. He is the one from whom ritual action arises and he pervades this whole world. By worshipping the Deity through the performance of his proper duty, a man achieves that perfect state.

47. Even though it may have faults, one's own dharma is still superior to accepting the dharma of another, even if it is perfectly observed. By performing the action prescribed in accordance with his inherent nature, a person never experiences contamination.

48. A person should never give up the action he is born to perform, Kaunteya. All endeavors are covered by some fault, as fire is covered by smoke.

49. His mind is detached from everything, he has conquered his own self, and he is free from hankering; it is by means of such renunciation that a person attains the highest success free from the results of action.

50. Now learn from me in brief, Kaunteya, how one who has achieved this success then attains Brahman, which is the culmination of realized knowledge.

51. It is by properly engaging his purified intellect, controlling himself by his resolve, renouncing the objects of the senses

such as sound, and setting aside both hankering and aversion;

52. Living in a deserted place, eating only a small amount, regulating his speech, body and mind, constantly dedicating himself to the Yoga of meditation and maintaining a mood of renunciation;

53. Giving up egotism, physical power, pride, desire, anger and any sense of possession, having no conception of "mine", and remaining always at peace; it is thus that he achieves the state of being that is Brahman.

54. Existing as Brahman, with his mind made tranquil, he neither laments nor hankers for anything. He is equal to all living beings. Such a person achieves the highest state of devotion to me.

55. And it is through this devotion that he gains knowledge of me, of my greatness and my true identity. When he thus properly understands me, he then immediately enters my being.

56. Always performing his prescribed duties while remaining dependent upon me, through my grace he attains the eternal, changeless position.

57. Mentally renouncing all your actions to me, dedicating yourself to me, and devoting yourself to the Buddhi Yoga, you should keep your mind always fixed on me.

58. Keeping your mind fixed on me, you will cross beyond all these difficulties through my grace. But if through pride you do not listen, you will perish.

59. If you surrender to your egotism and think, "I will not fight," this determination will be false and your inherent nature will exert its control over you.

60. Bound to your specific form action, Kaunteya, which arises

APPENDIX

from your inherent nature, you will be compelled to perform the action that because of illusion you do not wish to perform.

61. The Lord of all beings is situated in the region of the heart and he causes every being to revolve through life, mounted on the machine created by his mystical power (maya).

62. You should surrender to him with your entire being, Bharata, and then by his grace you will attain the highest position, which is absolute peace.

63. I have now revealed to you this wisdom, which is the deepest mystery. After fully considering what you have heard, you should then act as you see fit.

64. Now listen again to the ultimate teaching, which is the deepest mystery of all. You are very dear to me, this is certain, and therefore I will reveal this for your benefit.

65. Fix your mind on me, become my devotee, worship me and bow down to me. Then you will come to me, this is my certain promise for you are dear to me.

66. Abandoning all types of dharma take shelter with me alone. I will deliver you from all sins so do not be afraid.

67. You should not reveal these teachings to anyone who has no austerity or is bereft of devotion, nor to one who does not wish to hear it or who is envious of me.

68. But one who imparts this supreme mystery to my devotees after developing the highest devotion to me will come to me. There is no doubt about this.

69. There is no one among men who can perform a deed more pleasing to me than this and nor will there be any person more dear to me than he.

70. And if anyone studies this conversation between us based on dharma, then he worships me with the yajña of knowledge. That is my view.

71. Any man endowed with faith and free of malice who hears this discourse is liberated thereby and attains the auspicious worlds gained by those of righteous deeds.

72. Have you listened to this instruction with a focused mind, Partha? Is your confusion based on ignorance now dispelled, Dhanamjaya?

73. Arjuna said: The confusion is dispelled and through your grace I have regained my understanding. My doubts have vanished and I am now ready to act in accordance with your instruction.

74. Samjaya said: Thus I have heard this wonderful conversation between Vasudeva and the great soul who is Partha, which fills me with ecstasy.

75. It is through the grace of Vyasa that I have heard this supreme secret, this doctrine of Yoga that was revealed by Krishna himself who is the master of Yoga (yogeshvara).

76. O king, as I constantly recall this wonderful and sacred conversation between Keshava and Arjuna, I repeatedly experience this sense of ecstasy.

77. And as I repeatedly recall the magnificent form displayed by Hari, great is my sense of wonder, O king, and again and again I feel a thrill of delight.

78. Wherever there is Krishna, the master of Yoga, and wherever there is Partha who bears the bow, there will also be good fortune, victory, success and good judgment. That is my opinion.

THE SEVEN MAIN TEACHINGS OF BAHAGAVAD GITA

1. Dharma
2. Karma
3. Moksha
4. Bhakti and the Nature of God
5. Yoga
6. Ethical Conduct
7. The Three Gunas

DHARMA

For the *Bhagavad Gita*, dharma means both virtuous conduct and the social duties an individual is bound to perform in relation to his *varna* or social class. In Chapter 1, Arjuna argues that the death of family elders leads to a decline in family dharma while in Chapter 7 (v 12), Krishna identifies himself as desire but only when it does not contravene dharma. The main reference to dharma, however, is in relation to Krishna's insistence that Arjuna must fulfil the dharma of his social class, the *kshatriyas*, by waging war against wrongdoers. We first find this instruction in Chapter 2, verses 31-36. Moreover, the Karma Yoga that Krishna emphasizes in the opening chapters of the *Gita* is based on the idea that dharma or duty should be performed without desire for personal gain. In Chapter 18, the concept of dharma is revisited with some interesting refinements of the points made earlier. In vss41-44, the dharma of each *varna* is outlined and in verses 45-46 a link is made between dharma and *bhakti*, for dharmic duty is a means of worshipping God. It is therefore wrong for an individual to abandon his or her dharma; in any case dharma is not just a series of tasks one ought to perform it is a part of one's very nature. Hence for the *Gita* dharma is descriptive as well as prescriptive; it is not just what a person ought to do, it is a reflection of a person's inner nature (*sva-bhava*) generated as a result of past karma.

KARMA

The idea of good and bad fortune in this world being the result of previous actions, or karma, is fundamental to Indian religious thought and is more or less taken for granted in the *Bhagavad Gita*. Arjuna's reluctance to fight is based in part on his fear of the future results of sinful action; and in Chapter 14, Krishna relates the idea of karma to the influence of the three *gunas* over human action. The *Gita*, however, refines the doctrine of karma still further by insisting that it is the consciousness of the performer rather than the action itself that is the crucial factor. This again is related to the idea of Karma Yoga. In Chapter 4, it is explained that actions performed without selfish desire are *akarma* because they produce no reaction while even a failure to act produces a result if it is based on desire. This idea is taken up again in the first twenty verses or so of Chapter 18. Action, good or bad, produces future results and rebirth (rat race, within the box) in another body, and so one might think that *moksha*, release from rebirth (rat race, within the box), can be gained only by renouncing all action. The *Bhagavad Gita* teaches, however, that it is not the action itself that must be renounced but the selfish desire that prompts it. In this way the performance of dharmic duty becomes compatible with escaping from the cycle of good and bad karma.

MOKSHA

The *Bhagavad Gita* is essentially a *moksha shastra* as its main purpose is to teach its hearers how to gain release from rebirth (rat race, within the box). It is anxious to show that the quest for *moksha* need not necessarily involve giving up dharmic duty and for this reason it offers a Karma Yoga. In Chapter 6, the Dhyana Yoga is revealed as a spiritual practice that led to liberation (breakthrough) (breakthrough) from rebirth (rat race, within the box). And then in Chapters 7 to 12 we are shown that *moksha* is in fact a gift of grace granted by Krishna himself to the devotees whom he loves. This is revealed particularly in 7.14, 11.55, 12.6-7 and 18.66. While the *Gita* offers several different paths to *moksha*, including karma, *dhyana* and *bhakti*, it does not say a great deal about what *moksha* actually is or the form in which one exists in that state. There are many different phrases used by the *Gita* to refer to *moksha* but they do little more than to reveal that this is a state in which Krishna exists, that it is joyful and that it's free from any danger of a return to the state of existence in which rebirth (rat race, within the box) takes place. It is also clear from verses such as 8.15-16, 9.33 and 13.8 that the *Gita* regards this world as a place of suffering from which one should seek to escape.

BHAKTI AND THE NATURE OF GOD

There is a lot that can be written under this heading as it is a topic that the *Bhagavad Gita* deals with in some detail. In considering 'the nature of God' one might look at the avatar verses at the start of Chapter 4 and then the discussions in Chapter 7, Chapter 9 and the opening verses of Chapter 10. One might also consider the significance of the *vishva-rupa* revealed to Arjuna in Chapter 11. There is substantial evidence to suggest that the *Gita* regards *bhakti* as the best spiritual path for an aspirant to follow. In following the Karma Yoga and the Dhyana Yoga described in Chapter 6 one relies on one's own efforts to transform oneself through higher realization. It is clear, however, that Krishna himself grants *moksha* to his devotee as an act of divine grace. This is apparent from verses such as 7.14, 10.11, 12.6-7 and 18.66. Moreover, the *Bhagavad Gita* provides the foundation for the emotional forms of devotion that are so important in Hinduism today.

In Chapter 12, Krishna repeatedly refers to the mood of love that exists between himself and his devotee, using the word *priya* to make the point. So there really is a lot that can be said under this heading!

YOGA

The *Bhagavad Gita* uses the term Yoga for all the paths it recommends and this allows for a very broad definition. Here, however, it is probably a good idea to confine oneself to a narrower definition and look at the teachings it provides on the type of Yoga recommended by Patañjali in his *Yoga Sutras*. In Chapter 6 and again in Chapter 8, Krishna instructs Arjuna in techniques of meditation and inward contemplation. The important points to note here are the techniques recommended, the object of meditation and the reasons why this practice is suggested. It is clear that the Yoga taught by the *Gita* is intended to allow realization of the *atman* within one's own being and that this realization is a regarded as a means of transcending the conditions of life in this world. The techniques advocated involve *asana*, withdrawal of the senses from external objects and the regulation of the mind so that it can be fixed on a single point and maintained in that intense form of contemplation. It is also interesting to note Arjuna's response to this teaching, which we find in verses 33 and 34 of Chapter 6.

ETHICAL CONDUCT

Arjuna's initial objection to fighting rests substantially on his view that to do so would be *adharma*, a breach of his ethical code. In teaching a Karma Yoga, Krishna switches the focus away from the action itself toward the motive that prompts a person to perform it. Hence for Arjuna, killing those who oppose him is acceptable, providing his motive is not one of selfish desire. Here also Krishna reasserts the traditional notion of *varna-dharma*, insisting that it is Arjuna's duty to fight because of his social identity as a *kshatriya* or warrior. The *Bhagavad Gita* does not give lists of approved or forbidden acts, it is not a book of religious law, but it does provide lists of qualities that one should strive to incorporate into one's own character. In Chapter 13, verses 7 to 11 describe knowledge in terms of the qualities displayed by a person who possesses knowledge, though these seem to be more applicable to a person who has renounced the world to live as a monk. And in Chapter 16 we are given lists of qualities relating to persons who possess the nature of the gods and to those who possess the nature of the evil *asuras*. Here again, however, we have an interesting twist as in verse 5 Krishna tells Arjuna that he was born with the qualities of the gods, which, of course, raises questions as to whether morality is something one strives to achieve or is just something one is born with as a result of previous action.

THE THREE GUNAS

The idea that matter is pervaded by three fundamental qualities, *sattva*, *rajas* and *tamas*, is an important element of Samkhya philosophy and it is one that the *Bhagavad Gita* makes extensive use of, particularly in its later chapters. Chapter 13 emphasizes the division between *prakriti* and *purusha* (matter and spirit), but it is in Chapter 14 that we find an extensive analysis of the way in which these three *gunas* (literally strands or qualities) influence and shape the lives of living beings. In Chapter 17 and verses 18-40 of Chapter 18, Krishna uses the *gunas* as a basis for his discussion of different facets of human life including such categories as food, charity, austerity, knowledge, action and pleasure. He thereby demonstrates how the *gunas*are influential in shaping different areas of human life and also human nature. Ultimately, however, one who seeks *moksha* must go beyond all three *gunas*, even *sattva* which represents purity and goodness. Verses 25 and 26 of Chapter 14 make it clear that one who seeks the highest goal must become *gunatita*, completely beyond the range of the *gunas*.

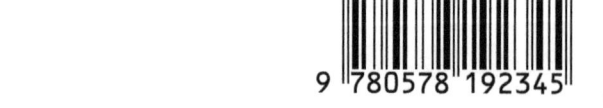

Lightning Source UK Ltd.
Milton Keynes UK
UKHW010103231019
352094UK00001B/68/P

9 780578 192345